Workbook

# Rau's Respiratory Care Pharmacology

*Seventh Edition*

**Douglas S. Gardenhire, EdD(c), RRT**
Director of Clinical Education
Division of Respiratory Therapy
School of Health Professions
College of Health and Human Sciences
Georgia State University
Atlanta, Georgia

**Robert J. Harwood, MSA, RRT-NPS**
Clinical Assistant Professor
Division of Respiratory Therapy
School of Health Professions
College of Health and Human Sciences
Georgia State University
Atlanta, Georgia

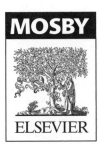

MOSBY

ELSEVIER

11830 Westline Industrial Drive
St. Louis, Missouri 63146

WORKBOOK FOR RAU'S RESPIRATORY CARE PHARMACOLOGY,      ISBN 978-0-323-04949-8
SEVENTH EDITION
**Copyright © 2008, 2002 by Mosby, Inc., an affiliate of Elsevier Inc.**

---

**Notice**

Knowledge and best practice in this field are constantly changing. As new research and experience broaden
our knowledge, changes in practice, treatment, and drug therapy may become necessary or appropriate.
Readers are advised to check the most current information provided (i) on procedures featured or (ii) by
the manufacturer of each product to be administered, to verify the recommended dose or formula, the
method and duration of administration, and contraindications. It is the responsibility of practitioners,
relying on their own experience and knowledge of the patient, to make diagnoses, to determine dosages
and the best treatment for each individual patient, and to take all appropriate safety precautions. To the
fullest extent of the law, neither the Publisher nor the Author assumes any liability for any injury and/or
damage to persons or property arising out of or related to any use of the material contained in this book.

The Publisher

---

**International Standard Book Number 978-0-323-04949-8**

*Managing Editor:* Mindy Hutchinson
*Associate Developmental Editor:* Christina Pryor
*Publishing Services Manager:* Pat Joiner-Myers
*Senior Project Manager:* Karen M. Rehwinkel

Working together to grow
libraries in developing countries

www.elsevier.com | www.bookaid.org | www.sabre.org

ELSEVIER    BOOK AID International    Sabre Foundation

Printed in The United States of America

Last digit is the print number:  9  8  7  6  5  4

# Contents

# 1 Introduction to Respiratory Care Pharmacology

## OBJECTIVES

*After answering the following questions, the reader should be able to:*

1. Define *pharmacology*
2. Define *drugs*
3. Describe how drugs are named
4. List the different sources of drug information
5. List the various sources used to manufacture drugs
6. Describe the process for drug approval in the United States
7. Define *orphan drugs*
8. Differentiate between prescription drugs and over-the-counter drugs
9. Apply the various abbreviations and symbols used in prescribing drugs
10. Describe the therapeutic purpose of each of the major aerosolized drug groups

## KEY TERMS AND DEFINITIONS

*Complete the following questions by writing the answer in the space provided.*

1. A chemical that changes an organism's function is called a _____.

2. The study of drugs (chemicals) is called _____.

3. The time course and disposition of a drug in the body, based on its absorption, distribution, metabolism, and elimination, is called _____.

4. The mechanism of drug action by which a drug molecule causes its effect in the body is called _____.

5. _____ _____ is a gram-negative organism and is primarily a nosocomial organism.

6. The study of toxic substances and their pharmacological actions, including antidotes and poison control, is called

   _____.

7. The name assigned to a chemical, when it appears that the chemical has therapeutic use and the manufacturer wishes to market the drug, is _____ _____.

8. A virus that causes the formation of syncytial masses in cells and may cause respiratory distress in young infants is called _____ _____ _____.

9. The name indicating a drug's chemical structure is _____ _____.

10. The art of treating disease with drugs is called _____.

*Complete the following by writing the answer in the space provided.*

11. A _____ name is given to an experimental chemical that shows promise as a drug.

12. The _____ name-brand name; proprietary name given to a drug by the manufacturer (*example:* trade names for ibuprofen include Advil and Motrin; Tylenol is a trade name for acetaminophen).

13. The _____ name indicates the drug's chemical structure.

14. The _____ name is what the generic name becomes once it receives official approval.

15. The _____ name is the nonproprietary name (*example:* ibuprofen; acetaminophen).

16. Fill in the following different names for the antiasthmatic drug zafirlukast.

    a. Chemical name _____

    b. Code name _____

    c. Official name _____

    d. Generic name _____

    e. Trade name _____

## SOURCES OF DRUG INFORMATION

*Complete the following questions by writing the answer in the space provided.*

17. What is an official source of information about drug standards if you want to obtain information about medications, dietary supplements, and medical devices? The U.S. Food and Drug Administration (FDA) considers this book the official standard for drugs marketed in the United States.

18. This reference source, commonly known as the PDR, has lots of color charts that identify drugs, lists manufacturers, and tells how the drugs work, when they're indicated and contraindicated, and possible side effects.

19. Another place to look is the American Society of Health-System Pharmacists' publication, called

    _____. This book gives more general information about classes of drugs (such as antibiotics and antidepressants).

## SOURCES OF DRUGS

*Complete the following questions by writing the answer in the space provided.*

20. Most of today's drugs come from chemicals, but _____, _____, and

    _____ also contain certain active ingredients for drugs.

21. In ancient times cromolyn sodium was used as a muscle relaxant, but the synthetic form today is an

    _____.

22. Poppies are well known for containing opium. No wonder Dorothy and Toto fall asleep in The

    _____ _____ _____.

## PROCESS OF DRUG APPROVAL IN THE UNITED STATES

It's time-consuming and expensive to get a drug approved in the United States. To make it worse, most chemicals that were identified as potential drugs (remember RT#007?) don't ever make it to the general clinical use stage.

*Complete the following questions by writing the correct term in the blank provided.*

23. Investigational New Drug (IND) Approval. Next, an IND application outlining plans for human studies must be submitted to the FDA. Human studies are done in three phases and take about 3 years to finish. In each phase include the study subjects.

    a. Phase 1: _____

    b. Phase 2: _____

    c. Phase 3: _____

24. A detailed reporting system is in place for _____ months to track any problems that arise with the drug's use.

New drugs are classified by the FDA with a number followed by a hyphen and a letter. Match each of the following letters with the correct definition by placing the letter of the best answer in the space provided.

25. _____ Important (significant) therapeutic gain over other drugs     A
        AA
26. _____ Modest therapeutic gain     B
        C
27. _____ Important therapeutic gain, indicated
    for a patient with AIDS; fast-track

28. _____ Little or no therapeutic gain

*After each question, provide the correct answer.*

29. List one advantage of orphan drugs.

30. List one disadvantage of orphan drugs.

## THE PRESCRIPTION

The prescription is the written order for a drug. It contains instructions for the pharmacist and the patient about how to make, dispense, and take the drug.

*Answer the following questions about the prescription.*

31. Name the six parts of a prescription.

   a. _____

   b. _____

   c. _____

   d. _____

   e. _____

   f. _____

32. Give an example of an over-the-counter (OTC) drug.

33. True or False: The physician must write on the prescription that it's okay to use the generic form of the drug.

## RESPIRATORY CARE PHARMACOLOGY: AN OVERVIEW

*Complete the following question by writing the correct terms in the blanks provided.*

Using Tables 1-2 and 1-3 in the textbook, provide the correct answers for the following questions.

34. List three advantages of aerosolized agents given by inhalation.

   a. _____

   b. _____

   c. _____

35. Fill in the blank sections of the following table.

| Drug Group | Therapeutic Purpose | Agent |
|---|---|---|
| Adrenergic | | Albuterol |
| Anticholinergic | Relaxation of bronchoconstriction | |
| Mucoactive | | Mucomyst |
| Corticosteroid | Reduction of airway inflammation | |
| Antiasthmatic | | |
| Antiinfective | Elimination of infective agents | |
| Surfactant | | Infasurf |

36. Match the following list of abbreviations with their meanings. These are used when writing prescriptions and in patient's hospital charts.

a. q4h _____

b. qd _____

c. bid _____

d. et _____

e. cc _____

f. gtt _____

g. IM _____

h. L _____

i. ml _____

j. po _____

k. q _____

l. prn _____

m. nebul _____

n. npo _____

o. qh _____

a drop
a spray
and
as needed
by mouth
cubic centimeter
every
every 2 hours
every 3 hours
every 4 hours
every day
every hour
every other day
four times daily
intramuscular
intravenous
liter
milliliter
nothing by mouth
three times daily
twice daily

p. qod _____

q. q3h _____

r. qid _____

s. q2h _____

t. tid _____

u. IV _____


## RELATED DRUG GROUPS IN RESPIRATORY CARE

*Complete the following questions by writing the answer in the space provided.*

37. Drugs used to treat infections, such as antibiotics and antifungal drugs, are called _____

_____.

38. These agents paralyze people and are used in critical care. An example of this type of drug is Pavulon.

_____ _____ _____.

39. A drug used to help reduce the effect of pain by affecting the central nervous system (*example:* morphine)

is called a(n) _____.

40. Drugs that treat dangerous cardiac dysrhythmias are called (*example:* lidocaine) _____.

41. These drugs, used to treat high blood pressure and chest pain, are called (*example:* β blockers, nitroglycerin)

_____ _____ _____.

42. These agents help to keep blood from clotting (*example:* heparin). _____

_____ _____.

43. In order to rid the body of excess body fluid (whether it's in the lungs, heart, etc.) a(n)

_____ would be administered.

44. Match the aerosolized drug group with their agent.

1. _____ dornase alfa

2. _____ zafirlukast

3. _____ beractant

4. _____ ribavirin

5. _____ beclomethasone dipropionate

6. _____ ipratropium bromide

7. _____ epinephrine

a. Antiinfective agent
b. Antiasthmatic agent
c. Mucoactive agent
d. Anticholinergic agent
e. Adrenergic agent
f. Corticosteroid
g. Exogenous surfactant

## NATIONAL BOARD FOR RESPIRATORY CARE–TYPE QUESTIONS

*Now that you've had a chance to review this material from the text, try these questions that follow.*
*When you're finished, check your responses with the answer key at the end of the book.*

1. Animal studies are designed to accomplish which of the following?
   a. General effect on the organism
   b. Effects on specific organs
   c. Toxicology studies
   d. All the above

2. Studies involving human subjects occur during which stage of the drug approval process?
   a. Chemical identification
   b. IND approval
   c. NDA
   d. Internal review

3. Which of the following is the generic name for the antiasthmatic drug Accolate?
   a. Proventil
   b. Zafirlukast
   c. ICI 204,219
   d. ED-AA

4. If you are looking up a drug in a reference source that has color charts that identify drugs, lists manufacturers, and tells how the drugs work, you are looking in the
   a. Hospital Formulary
   b. Hospital Reference Source
   c. Physician's Desk Reference
   d. Drug Handbook

5. Which of the following is *not* an advantage of aerosolized agents by inhalation?
   a. Aerosol doses are larger than those used for the same purpose and given systemically
   b. Fewer side effects than those given systemically
   c. More rapid onset of action
   d. Drug delivery is targeted to the respiratory system and is painless

6. An order has been written for a patient to receive an aerosolized bronchodilator tid. This would indicate the patient should receive the treatment
   a. Four times a day
   b. Three times a day
   c. Once a day
   d. Every 3 hours

7. An agent that will relax bronchial smooth muscle and reduce airway resistance to improve ventilatory flow rate in COPD and asthma is
   a. Adrenergic
   b. Corticosteroid
   c. Anticholinergic
   d. Mucoactive

8. A patient has been ordered to receive a corticosteroid. This would indicate the patient has a need for
   a. Bronchial smooth muscle relaxation
   b. Thinning of mucus
   c. Increase in lung compliance
   d. Reduction and control of inflammatory response in the airway

9. This is an agent that is used to rid the body of excess fluid that may accumulate in the lungs.
   a. Antiinfective
   b. Antithrombolytic
   c. Diuretic
   d. Anticoagulant

10. As you enter a patient's room you notice a sign above the bed that reads "NPO." This would indicate
    a. Administer medications by mouth only
    b. Administer drugs by IV only
    c. Nothing by mouth
    d. No needle sticks

# 2 Principles of Drug Action

## CHAPTER OBJECTIVES

*After answering the following questions, the reader should be able to:*

1. Define the *drug administration phase*
2. Describe the various routes of administration available
3. Define the *pharmacokinetic phase*
4. Discuss the key factors in the pharmacokinetic phase (e.g., absorption, distribution, metabolism, and elimination)
5. Describe the first-pass effect
6. Differentiate between systemic and inhaled drugs in relation to the pharmacokinetic phase
7. Explain the L/T ratio
8. Define the *pharmacodynamic phase*
9. Discuss the importance of structure–activity relations
10. Discuss the role of drug receptors
11. Discuss the importance of dose–response relations
12. Describe the importance of pharmogenetics

## KEY TERMS AND DEFINITIONS

*Match the following definitions with their terms.*

1. _____ A rapid decrease in response to a drug.

2. _____ A drug interaction that occurs from combined drug effects that are greater than if the drugs were given alone.

3. _____ Drug administration in any way other than by the intestine, most commonly by intravenous, intramuscular, or subcutaneous injection.

4. _____ Taking a substance, typically in the form of gases, fumes, vapors, mists, aerosols, or dusts, into the body by breathing in.

5. _____ Administration of a drug by use of the intestine.

6. _____ Difference between the minimal therapeutic and toxic concentrations of the a drug; the smaller the difference the greater chance the drug will be toxic.

7. _____ A chemical or drug that binds to a receptor and creates an effect on the body.

8. _____ An abnormal or unexpected reaction to a drug, other than an allergic reaction, as compared with the predicted effect.

a. Parenteral
b. Transdermal
c. Inhalation
d. Enteral
e. Lung availability/systemic availability (L/T ratio)
f. Therapeutic index (TI)
g. Agonist
h. Synergistic effect
i. Idiosyncratic effect
j. Tachyphylaxis

9. _____ Amount of drug that is made available
out of the total available to the lung.

10. _____ Use of a patch on the skin to deliver a
drug.

## THE DRUG ADMINISTRATION PHASE

The drug administration phase describes the method by which a drug dose is made available to the body. The two key topics here include drug dosage form and route of administration.

*Complete the following questions by writing the correct term in the blank provided.*

11. Tablets, capsules, and injectable solutions are examples of _____

_____ forms.

12. Oral, injection, and inhalation are examples of the _____ _____

_____.

13. List the five ways that a drug can be administered and give one example of a common drug formulation.

| Administration of Drug | Common Drug Formulation |
|---|---|
| a. _____ | a. _____ |
| b. _____ | b. _____ |
| c. _____ | c. _____ |
| d. _____ | d. _____ |
| e. _____ | e. _____ |

## THE PHARMACOKINETIC PHASE

To understand how a drug works from the time it's given to the time it takes effect, you need to understand the three phases that it progresses through.

*Complete the following questions by writing the correct term in the blank provided.*

14. How the drug gets absorbed, distributed, metabolized, and eliminated is the _____ phase.

15. How the drug causes an effect in the body is the _____ phase.

16. List the five layers of the lower respiratory tract that a drug must traverse before reaching the blood stream for distribution into the body.

a. _____

b. _____

c. _____

d. _____

e. _____

## Absorption

For a drug to work, it must be absorbed. A drug is absorbed in four ways: lipid diffusion, carrier-mediated transport, aqueous diffusion, and pinocytosis.

*Fill in the blank with the type of absorption.*

17. This type of diffusion occurs in _____ compartments of the body, such as interstitial spaces or inside a cell.

18. _____ diffusion occurs across epithelial cells with lipid membranes. For a drug to be distributed in the body, it must cross the many epithelial membranes that have lipid membranes before it reaches the target organ. Nonionized drugs are lipid soluble; ionized forms of drugs are water soluble (lipid insoluble). Nonionized or lipid-soluble drugs are well absorbed into the blood stream and across the blood–brain barrier.

19. _____ _____ transport occurs by special membrane-embedded carrier molecules transporting substances across membranes.

20. _____ is the incorporation of a substance into a cell by a process of membrane engulfment and transport of the substance to the cell interior in vesicles, thereby allowing translocation across a membrane barrier.

21. This term is used to indicate the proportion of drug that reaches the systemic circulation. For example, if oral morphine has a _____ of 0.24 that means only one-fourth of the drug reaches the systemic circulation.

22. Which of the following drug types is best absorbed into the blood stream? Circle as many as are correct.
    Nonionized
    Water soluble
    Ionized
    Lipid soluble

## Distribution

To be effective, a drug must have a certain concentration. This concentration is determined partly by the rate of absorption versus the rate of elimination and partly by the volume of drug. A drug will be distributed to one or more body compartments.

23. List the approximate volume in liters of each of the following major body compartments.

| Compartment | Volume (L) |
|---|---|
| a. Vascular (blood) | _____ |
| b. Interstitial fluid | _____ |
| c. Intracellular fluid | _____ |
| d. Fat (adipose tissue) | _____ |

You can determine the drug concentration from a blood sample. But because the drug may be distributed in a compartment other than the vascular compartment, the calculated volume of distribution can be larger than the blood volume. For this reason, the volume of distribution is referred to as the *apparent volume of distribution (AVD)*.

You can use $V_D$ to determine an appropriate dose for a given therapeutic level, if you rearrange the equation.

Using the example from text: To produce a theophylline concentration of 10 mg/L, with a $V_D$ of 35 L, what dose do you give?

$$V_D = \text{drug amount} / \text{plasma concentration}$$

$$\text{Amount (dose)} = V_D \times \text{concentration}$$

$$\text{Does} = (35L)(10mg/L) = 350 \text{ mg}$$

24. See how clear it is! Let's give it a try. What's the AVD (in liters) if I give a 100-mg dose of a drug whose concentration is 5 mg/L?

## Metabolism

*Complete the following questions by writing the correct term in the blank provided.*

25. Phase 1 metabolism is where the drug is converted to a more _____ -soluble form by enzymes within the liver, allowing the drug to be more easily excreted.

26. The main organ for drug metabolism is the _____.

27. Inhibition or increase of enzymes within the liver can occur with _____ of drugs metabolized by the liver.

28. Enzyme induction may cause drugs to have a shorter _____-_____ and require adjustment of dosages.

29. If a drug is highly metabolized by the liver, most of the drug's effect will be lost in passing into the liver, before it

   even gets to the general circulation. This clinically important effect is called the _____-

   _____ effect.

## Elimination

*Complete the following questions by writing the correct term in the blank provided.*

30. The primary site for drug excretion is the _____.

31. The measure of a body's ability to rid itself of a drug is called _____.

   _____ clearance gives an indication of the quantity of drug removed from the body over a given time. It can be used to estimate the rate at which drug must be replaced to maintain a steady plasma level.

32. The time required for the plasma concentration of a drug to decrease by one-half is called the

   _____ _____-_____.

33. True or False: Drugs with a short half-life must be given more frequently to maintain plasma levels.

34. True or False: Drugs with a long half-life take longer to reach steady-state levels but do not have to be given as frequently.

35. To achieve a steady level of drug in the body, dosing must equal the rate of _____.

**12**

The concentration of a drug in the body over time can be graphed as a time–effect curve as seen in Figure 2-5 of the textbook. The curve's shape describes a *bioavailability profile*, which can tell you whether the dose you've given is enough to produce a therapeutic effect.

*Using Figure 2-5 in the textbook, provide the correct answer to the following questions. Consider drugs A, B, and C to be bronchodilators.*

36. Which drug would be considered fast acting but of short duration? _____

37. If a person needed a long-acting drug for nighttime duration, which one would meet the person's needs?

    _____

38. Which bronchodilator drug would be useful for maintenance therapy and a duration of action of 4-6 hours?

    _____

## Pharmacokinetics of Inhaled Aerosol Drugs

*After each question, provide the correct answer(s) or fill in the blank(s).*

39. What is the difference between a local drug effect and a systemic drug effect?

40. Give an example of a drug that causes a local effect and a drug that causes a systemic effect.

41. When delivering a drug by inhalation both _____ and _____ absorption occurs.

42. What percentage of an inhaled aerosol is swallowed?

43. How much of it gets to the lungs?

44. How much aerosol impacts in the mouth and contributes to the amount reaching the stomach?




45. List one advantage of a local versus a systemic effect when administering a drug in this way.




46. What could be attached to a metered-dose inhaler (MDI) to increase the amount of drug reaching the lungs?




47. True or False: If a swallowed aerosol drug is highly metabolized by the liver, then the systemic effects will be due to lung absorption.

48. Lung availability/total systemic availability (L/T) basically tells how efficient _____ delivery is into the lung.

49. List four factors that increase the L/T ratio with inhaled drugs. What does each factor have in common?

   a. _____

   b. _____

   c. _____

   d. _____

50. True or False: The L/T ratio also determines whether systemic toxicity or side effects will occur.




## THE PHARMACODYNAMIC PHASE

Remember this phase? *Pharmacodynamics* describes the mechanisms of drug action (how it works), that is, the way the drug causes its effect on the body.

*Complete the following question by writing the correct term in the blank provided.*

51. For a drug to cause any effect in the body, it must combine with a _____.

**Structure–Activity Relations**

The drug and the receptor must be structurally similar for matching to occur. The structure–activity relation (SAR) describes the relationship between the chemical structure of the drug and its clinical effect. Take isoproterenol and albuterol as examples. They have similar chemical structures, so they will both match to airway receptors. But the chemical structures are different enough to make a clinical difference—isoproterenol will also match with receptors found in the heart, which may cause increased heart rate in patients who receive this drug. Albuterol has a longer side chain (part of its chemical structure), which makes it a more selective "key," so that it only matches with receptors in the airways.

*Circle the correct answer.*

52. The more complex the chemical structure of a drug, the (more, fewer) receptors it will match.

**Nature and Type of Drug Receptors**

Most drug receptors are proteins whose shape and electrical charge make them a match for a drug's shape and charge. For this "matching" to occur, a process called *transmembrane signaling* must occur. This can happen in one of four different ways.

1. Lipid-soluble drugs cross the cell membrane and act on intracellular receptors to initiate a drug response. Corticosteroids work this way.

2. The drug attaches to the extracellular part of the receptor, which projects into the cell cytoplasm (a "transmembrane protein"), and activates an enzyme system that produces the desired effect. Insulin is an example of this process.

3. The drug attaches to a receptor on the surface of the membrane, which opens an ion channel for the drug to move through. Acetylcholine receptors on skeletal muscle work this way.

4. The drug attaches to a transmembrane receptor that is hooked up to an intracellular enzyme by something called a G protein. β-Adrenergic agents work via this process. There is a G protein ($G_s$) that stimulates an enzyme called adenylyl cyclase This causes bronchodilation. Another G protein ($G_i$) inhibits adenylyl cyclase, which has the opposite effect on bronchial smooth muscle.

*Complete the following questions by writing the answer in the space provided.*

53. At present, drugs having the greatest relevance to respiratory therapy act through _____

    _____.

54. An increase in _____ protein stimulates _____ causing

    bronchodilation. This is an example of _____.

**Dose–Response Relations**

*After reading the following material, complete the following questions in the space provided.*

- The body's response to a drug is directly proportional to the drug's concentration.
- As more drug is given, more receptors are occupied, so drug effect will increase up to the point where all receptor sites are occupied. The dose at which 50% of the maximal response occurs is called the *effective dose* ($ED_{50}$). This refers to a drug's *potency*.
- The *maximal effect* of a drug is the greatest response that can be produced by the drug so that even at a higher dose, you won't get any more response.
- The more potent a drug is, the less it takes to produce 50% of the maximal response. For example, if drug A can elicit 50% maximal response with 2 mg, but it takes 4 mg of drug B to do the same thing, drug A is twice as potent as drug B. Two drugs might have the same potency but different maximal effects.

55. The body's response to a drug is directly proportional to the drug's _____.

56. The _____ _____ of a drug is the greatest response that can be produced by the drug so that even at a higher dose you won't get any more response.

The *therapeutic index* (TI) is also based on the dose–response curve of a drug. The difference here is, you're looking for an all-or-nothing response from subjects—they either improve or they don't. Improvement is quantified on the basis of the $ED_{50}$, the dose at which half the test subjects improve. On the flip side, the lethal dose ($LD_{50}$) represents the dose that will be lethal to 50% of the population of test subjects. Needless to say, animals are used for the test population! Now for the definition you've been waiting for:

$$TI = LD_{50}/ED_{50}$$

TI gives you an idea of how safe the drug is. The smaller the TI, the more dangerous the drug ($ED_{50}$ and $LD_{50}$ are closer, so don't screw up your patient's prescription!). For example, penicillin has a high TI (about 100)—lethal and effective doses are really far apart, so it's a safe drug. Digitalis, on the other hand, has a TI of about 1.5, so be careful.

57. Which drug is more potent? Drug A ($ED_{50} = 10$ mg) or drug B ($ED_{50} = 6$ mg)?

58. The TI of a drug is 3. This drug is relatively (safe, dangerous).

59. A drug that binds to a receptor (affinity) and causes a response (efficacy) is called a(n) _____.

60. True or False: A full agonist gives you a greater maximal response than a partial agonist.

61. Does this mean that a partial agonist has less affinity or less efficacy?

An *antagonist* can bind to the receptor but doesn't cause a response—it has affinity but no efficacy. Worse yet, an antagonist can hog the receptor site and keep other drugs from reaching the receptor site.

62. Affinity + efficacy = _____

63. Affinity – efficacy = _____

Positive interactions between drugs fall into three categories: synergism, additive, and potentiation.

64. Two drugs whose maximal effect is the sum of the effect of each drug alone is an example of

_____.

65. Two drugs having an effect greater than the sum of the effect of each drug alone is an example

of _____.

66. Match the following drug interactions with their mathematical definition:

   a. $1 + 0 = 2 =$      Synergism
   b. $1 + 1 = 3 =$      Potentiation
   c. $1 + 1 = 2 =$      Additivity

67. A special case of synergism, in which one drug has no effect but can increase the activity of the other drug, is an

   example of _____.

Terms that describe an individual's response to a drug include *hypersensitivity, tolerance, tachyphylaxis,* and *idiosyncratic.*

68. A drug that has the opposite effect, an unusual effect, or no effect compared with the effect it's supposed to have

    is said to be _____.

69. The term _____ describes an allergic or immune-related response to a drug that can be

    quite serious, even requiring ventilatory support.

70. The term _____ describes a decreasing intensity of response to a drug over time; over time

    more of the drug is required to produce the same effect.

71. The term _____ describes a rapid decrease in responsiveness to a drug.

## PHARMACOGENETICS

The well-described variations between patients in their responses to drugs are being increasingly traced to hereditary differences. The study of these genetic or hereditary differences is referred to as *pharmacogenetics*.

*Provide the answer to the following question.*

72. When do these genetic or hereditary variations manifest themselves?

## NATIONAL BOARD FOR RESPIRATORY CARE—TYPE QUESTIONS

And now, the moment you've been waiting for—20 NBRC-type questions! Yes, the answers are provided at the end of the book, but don't look until you have done all 20!

1. Which of the following describes what a drug does to the body?
   a. Pharmaceutical
   b. Pharmacokinetics
   c. Pharmacodynamics
   d. Pharmacongalines

2. Which of the following is the only route of administration that cannot exert a local effect?
   a. Topical
   b. Oral
   c. Parenteral
   d. Inhalation

3. Which type of drug crosses the blood–brain barrier most easily?
   I. Nonionized
   II. Ionized
   III. Lipid soluble
   IV. Water soluble
      a. I and III
      b. I and IV
      c. II and III
      d. II and IV

4. Which of the following is the main site of drug metabolism?
   a. Kidney
   b. Stomach
   c. Lung
   d. Liver

5. Which of the following is the main site of drug elimination?
   a. Intestine
   b. Stomach
   c. Kidney
   d. Liver

6. If a drug is administered more frequently than the half-life of the drug, which of the following may result?
   a. Synergy
   b. Accumulation
   c. Elimination
   d. Clearance

7. A patient has been taking a drug for several months; lately the patient requires more of the drug to produce the same effect. This is called
   a. Tolerance
   b. Hypersensitivity
   c. Tachyphylaxis
   d. Immunity

8. Inhaled aerosols used in the treatment of pulmonary disease are intended to exert what effect on the lung?
   a. Local
   b. Systemic
   c. Kinetic
   d. Dynamic

9. The drug dose at which 50% of its maximal response occurs is termed the $ED_{50}$. This refers to what aspect of the drug?
   a. Maximal effect
   b. Half-life
   c. Potency
   d. Bioavailability

10. Which of the following terms is used to describe what happens when an individual experiences less response to a drug over time?
    a. Hypersensitivity
    b. Idiosyncratic
    c. Toxicity
    d. Tolerance

11. For any drug to cause any effect in the body it must combine with which of the following?
    a. Target organ
    b. Another carrier drug
    c. Receptor
    d. Blood cell

12. Which of the following is the primary site for drug excretion?
    a. Liver
    b. Kidney
    c. Small intestine
    d. Large intestine

13. On the basis of Figure 2-5 (the time–effect curve in the textbook), which drug(s) would be considered long-acting for nighttime duration?
    a. Drug C only
    b. Drug A only
    c. Drug B only
    d. Drugs A and B

14. When delivering a drug by inhalation what percentage of the aerosol gets into the lung from most common aerosol devices?
    a. 10%
    b. 25%
    c. 20%
    d. 30%

15. Devices for administration of inhaled drugs include which of the following?
    I. Metered dose inhaler (MDI)
    II. Dry powder inhaler (DPI)
    III. Pneumatic nebulizer
    IV. Ultrasonic nebulizer
        a. I and II
        b. II and III
        c. II, III, and IV
        d. I, II, III, and IV

16. What could be done to increase the L/T ratio of an inhaled medication?
    a. Instruct the patient to breath fast and shallow.
    b. Use inhaled drugs with low first-pass metabolism.
    c. Use a reservoir device or holding chamber with an MDI.
    d. Instruct the patient to breath slowly when using a DPI.

17. Which of the following is a drug that binds to a receptor and causes a response?
    a. Agonist
    b. Efficist
    c. Additive
    d. Antagonist

18. The effect of two drugs being greater than the sum of the effect of each drug describes _____.
    a. Potentiation
    b. Additive
    c. Double whammy
    d. Synergism

19. If a patient requires more of a drug to produce the same effect it is said that the patient has built up

    _____ to the drug.
    a. Hypersensitivity
    b. Tolerance
    c. Tachyphylaxis
    d. Idiosyncracy

20. At present drugs having the greatest relevance to respiratory therapy act through which of the following receptors?
    a. Protein
    b. Enzymatic
    c. Intracellular
    d. Intranodal

R.E. is a 24-year-old who has been brought to the emergency room by his wife after having a high fever with shaking chills for the past 24 hours. R.E. states that he has had bronchitis for the past couple of weeks. He says that he is short of breath; his respiratory rate is 32 breaths/min; his heart rate is 108 beats/min. Auscultation reveals bilateral crackles in the lower lobes, with bilateral wheezing heard on inspiration. After examining him, both you and the physician agree that R.E. probably has pneumonia. R.E. will need a bronchodilator for the wheezing and antibiotics for the pneumonia.

1. Which route(s) of administration would be best to deliver the bronchodilator and antibiotics?

2. What drug would be best for his symptom of bilateral wheezing on inspiration?

R.E. has been admitted to the hospital and it is now day 2. He has been receiving albuterol treatments by small volume nebulizer and he is feeling much better. His respiratory rate is 18 breaths/min; his heart rate is 84 beats/min. The bilateral wheezing has been reduced and now there is a slight wheeze present bilaterally. R.E. comments that a lot of the medicine seems to be going out into the air and that he can taste it in the back of his throat. He asks you how much of the stuff really makes it into his lungs.

3. What do you tell him?

The doctor has ordered albuterol MDI to be used at home. You suggest that R.E. should also use a spacer device with the MDI. The doctor doesn't understand why the spacer device should also be used.

4. What would you tell the doctor?

# 3 | Administration of Aerosolized Agents

## CHAPTER OBJECTIVES

*After answering the following questions, the reader should be able to:*

1. Define aerosol therapy
2. Select an appropriate aerosol medication nebulizer on the basis of particle size distributions
3. Discuss aerosol particle size and deposition in the lungs
4. Differentiate between the types of aerosol devices
5. Describe the clinical applications of aerosol devices
6. Recommend the use of various aerosol devices

## KEY TERMS AND DEFINITIONS

*Complete the following questions by writing the answer in the space provided.*

1. The amount of solution that remains in the reservoir of a small volume nebulizer (SVN) once sputtering begins,

   causing a decrease in nebulization, is called the _____.

2. Testing in a laboratory is called _____ testing.

3. The diameter of a unit-density spherical particle having the same terminal settling velocity as the measured particle

   is the _____ _____ _____

   _____ .

4. A liquefied gas (e.g., Freon) propellant used to administer medication from a metered dose inhaler (MDI) is called

   a(n) _____.

5. An aerosol generator is also known as a(n) _____.

6. A nontoxic liquefied gas propellant used to administer medication from an MDI is a(n) _____

   _____.

7. An add-on device or extension for administration of a drug from an MDI is known as a(n)

   _____. It describes both a spacer and a valved holding chamber.

8. A simple tube that contains an aerosol cloud emitted from an MDI is called a(n) _____.
   Its function is to keep the MDI spray away from the mouth.

9. The process of particles depositing out of suspension to remain in the lung is called _____.

10. A spacer device with the addition of a one-way valve(s) to contain and hold the aerosol cloud until inspiration

    occurs is called a(n) _____ _____ _____.

11. The depth within the lung reached by particles is referred to as _____.

12. The tendency of aerosol particles to remain in suspension is described as _____.

## AEROSOL THERAPY

Before we get into the nitty-gritty of aerosol drugs, let's define aerosol therapy—it's the delivery of aerosol particles to the respiratory tract for therapeutic purposes.

*Complete the following questions by writing the answer in the space provided.*

13. What are three reasons for using aerosol therapy?

    a. _____

    b. _____

    c. _____

14. What are three advantages and three disadvantages seen with aerosol delivery of drugs?

| Advantages | Disadvantages |
|---|---|
| a. _____ | a. _____ |
| b. _____ | b. _____ |
| c. _____ | c. _____ |

## PHYSICAL PRINCIPLES OF INHALED AEROSOL DRUGS

*Complete the following questions by writing the answer in the space provided.*

15. For pulmonary diagnostic and therapeutic applications, the particle size range of interest is

    _____ μm.

16. Older aerosol-generating devices had an efficiency of 10% to 15% (only this much reached the respiratory tract).

    Newer devices have an efficiency of _____ % to _____ %.

17. Aerosol particles produced for inhalation into the lungs by MDIs, nebulizers, and dry powder inhalers (DPIs)

    come in many sizes—they're _____ or _____.

18. True or False: Aerosol particles are basically spherical.

19. You need to know what size the aerosol particles are, so that you can determine whether or not they'll make it into the airways or lung. The particle size above and below which 50% of the mass of the particles is found (i.e., the size that

    evenly divides the mass of the particles in the distribution) is called the _____

    _____ _____ _____ or MMAD.

20. The _____ of aerosol particles, or MMAD, is one of the most important factors in determining whether an aerosol will deposit in the lung.

21. The MMAD of aerosol particles that deposit in the nose and mouth is 10–15 μm. This size particle might be good

for _____ sprays.

22. How about the upper airways and early airway generations? Aerosol particles with an MMAD range of

_____ are lost there.

23. Aerosol particles with an MMAD range of _____ can make it to the lower respiratory tract. This is the appropriate size for the bronchoactive drugs that we use today.

24. Delivery of aerosols in the range of _____ is intended for the terminal airways and alveolar region. For example, an MMAD of 1 to 2 μm is suggested for peripheral deposition of the antiinfective drug pentamidine.

Particle size (MMAD) is not the only influence on where aerosol particles deposit in the lung; some aerosol generators are better suited than others for upper or lower airway delivery. For example, a respiratory department has ordered two types of SVN. One produces particles with an MMAD of 3.4 μm and the other produces an MMAD of 7.9 μm.

25. Which SVN would you use for a patient with expiratory wheezing primarily in the lower lung fields?

26. Which SVN would you use for a child with upper airway stridor from croup?

So what's the take-home message? Look at the MMAD or particle size that the aerosol generator will deliver and determine whether it will be better suited for delivery of aerosol particles to the upper or lower airway.

27. What are three factors that influence aerosol deposition in the lung?

a. _____, a function of particle size and velocity

b. _____, a function of particle size and time

c. _____, a function of time and random molecular motion

28. How much aerosol actually gets to the lung periphery also depends on the patient's _____ pattern.

29. On the basis of the three factors that influence aerosol deposition (see question 27), write down step-by-step instructions that you would give when instructing a patient on how to breathe during their medical nebulizer treatment?

30. Inhaled aerosol drugs are not only heterodisperse in size but readily absorb moisture; in other words, they are

_____. This leads to an increase in particle size, resulting in less aerosol delivery.

## AEROSOL DEVICES FOR DRUG DELIVERY

*Complete the following questions by writing the answer in the space provided.*

31. What is the difference between an ultrasonic nebulizer (USN) and an SVN?

32. On the basis of Box 3-2 and Box 3-3 in the textbook, identify which nebulizer, a portable USN or an SVN, would be best for the given situation of the individual needing aerosol therapy.

a. Older patient debilitated and in acute distress: _____

b. A person who travels extensively: _____

c. Unsure if drug will degrade with use of the nebulizer: _____

33. What is the purpose of the thumb control on an SVN?

34. How would you instruct a patient to use the thumb control during an SVN treatment?

35. Circle the correct answer: Because of significant evaporation of aqueous solution, drug solute can become (increasingly/decreasingly) concentrated.

36. True or False: Small volume nebulizers do not nebulize well when the volume in the reservoir is < 0.5 ml.

37. True or False: Adding diluent does not alter the amount of drug (dose) but simply expands the solution volume.

38. True or False: When sputtering of the nebulized medication occurs, shaking or agitating the reservoir will significantly increase drug solution delivery.

39. True or False: If the dead volume is not discarded and the reservoir rinsed an increasingly concentrated solution and drug dose could be administered with subsequent treatments.

40. For efficient operation and relatively brief treatments (≤5 minutes) a filling volume of _____ is recommended.

41. According to Figure 3-6 in the textbook, flow rate will decrease particle size, shifting the

_____ lower.

42. With a filling volume of 3–5 ml the flow rate should be between _____ and

_____.

43. An SVN can be powered by either _____ or _____.

44. Now that you know all the characteristics of the perfect nebulizer, fill in the following:

   a. Filling volume: _____

   b. Treatment time: _____

   c. Flow rate: _____

   d. Gas source: _____

45. Figure 3-7 in the textbook shows a comparison of three different types of SVN. Which of the three would have reduced ambient loss of aerosol and make more aerosol available to the patient. Why?

46. What are the five components of a metered dose inhaler (MDI)?

   a. _____

   b. _____

   c. _____

   d. _____

   e. _____

47. Chlorofluorocarbon (CFC) propellant is being replaced by _____ propellant.

To summarize: MDIs are effective because they are portable and small, deliver aerosol drugs as efficiently as an SVN (10%-15% of drug is delivered), and don't require much time per treatment. On the other hand, use of MDIs requires some coordination, it's difficult to tell when the canister is empty, a few patients may have a bad reaction to the propellant, and CFCs are released into the atmosphere.

48. The most common problem associated with MDI use is _____–

    _____ incoordination.

49. True or False: Storing a CFC propellant MDI canister of albuterol in a valve-up position will help reduce loss of dose (drug content in valve).

50. True or False: An MDI canister should not be shaken before the first actuation after the canister has been left to stand, in order to assure optimal dose discharge from the valve.

51. True or False: Wait 1-5 minutes between puffs of a bronchodilator so that the dose output is not reduced and to improve distribution of inhaled drug.

52. True or False: If an MDI hasn't been used for days or weeks, propellant may be lost. Without propellant, little or no drug will be discharged. If the MDI hasn't been used for a long time, it should be shaken and a waste discharge should be given to prime the valve with drug and propellant.

53. True or False: If a patient can't coordinate actuation and inspiration of an MDI, using an open-mouth technique, then a closed-mouth technique should be used.

54. An extension device such as a spacer or holding chamber should be used with what type of drug to reduce

    oropharyngeal impaction? _____

55. List three ways that valved holding chambers increase drug delivery.

    a. _____

    b. _____

    c. _____

56. Electrostatic charge on holding chambers can _____ drug delivery. If your patient is using a holding chamber at home you can instruct the patient to wash the spacer with standard household

    _____, which will reduce this charge.

57. What is a dry powder inhaler (DPI)?

58. The flow rate needed to disperse the drug of a dry powder inhaler is _____.

59. Once the dry powder device is activated and the drug is exposed the patient should not

    _____ into the device before inhaling.

## CLINICAL APPLICATION OF AEROSOL DELIVERY DEVICES

*Identify each of the following statements as either true or false.*

60. True or False: For treatment of adult and pediatric patients in the emergency department (ED), an MDI with a holding chamber and a nebulizer are equally effective.

61. True or False: It is better to use an MDI with a holding chamber, or an SVN, to deliver a short-acting $\beta_2$ agonist in the hospital than a DPI.

62. True or False: There are greater changes in lung function and asthma scores with the use of continuous nebulizer delivery of $\beta_2$ agonist than with the use of intermittent nebulizer delivery.

63. True or False: For children or adults being mechanically ventilated there is no difference between an MDI with a holding chamber and an SVN when administering aerosolized $\beta_2$ agonist.

64. True or False: The same clinical outcome is seen in adult asthmatic patients when using a DPI or an MDI with holding chamber.

65. True or False: To administer an equipotent dose of albuterol from an MDI and an SVN, the number of puffs from the albuterol MDI must be decreased. (Remember: The amount of bronchodilation obtained is a function of the dose of drug given rather than the way it is delivered.)

## AGE GUIDELINES FOR USE OF AEROSOL DEVICES

Age is an important factor to consider when selecting an aerosol delivery device.

66. Match the following aerosol systems to the appropriate age.

    1. _____ SVN

    2. _____ MDI

    3. _____ MDI with reservoir

    4. _____ MDI with reservoir and mask

    5. _____ MDI with endotracheal tube (ETT)

    6. _____ Breath-actuated MDI

    7. _____ DPI

    a. > 5 years of age
    b. ≥ neonate
    c. > 4 years
    d. ≤ 2 years
    e. ≤ 4 years

## ENDOTRACHEAL TUBE ADMINISTRATION

Aerosolized drug delivery commonly occurs with intubated neonates and adults. Evaluation of aerosol delivery is complicated by the number of variables introduced if the patient is undergoing mechanical ventilation and by the difficulty in quantifying drug delivery accurately. There are many variables with administration of aerosol drug through an endotracheal tube (ETT) to ventilated subjects with either SVN or MDI aerosol administration.

67. List three variables present when administering aerosol drug by SVN or MDI to intubated, mechanically ventilated patients.

**SVN**

a. _____

b. _____

c. _____

**MDI**

a. _____

b. _____

c. _____

68. Pediatric patients receiving aerosolized medications while undergoing mechanical ventilation may have a lower

percentage of drug delivered because of the _____ _____ being narrower.

69. To improve aerosol delivery, place the nebulizer _____ cm from the endotracheal tube on the inspiratory side of the patient circuit.

70. The _____–_____ _____ should be bypassed when delivering aerosolized medication to a patient receiving mechanical ventilation.

71. The use of a less dense gas, such as a _____–_____ mixture, can increase particle deposition.

72. When using an MDI, timing the actuation of the aerosol device with precise inspiration by the ventilator may

increase drug delivery by _____.

## NATIONAL BOARD FOR RESPIRATORY CARE–TYPE QUESTIONS

Now it's time once again for the NBRC-type questions.

1. Aerosol therapy is used for all but which of the following purposes?
   a. Humidification of inspired gases
   b. Improving mobilization and clearance of secretions
   c. Augmenting alveolar ventilation
   d. Delivery of medication

2. Which of the following are advantages of delivering medication using the aerosol versus systemic route of administration?
   I. Smaller doses are required.
   II. Onset of action is quicker.
   III. Side effects are fewer.
   IV. Drug delivery is targeted to the respiratory system.
       a. I, II, III, and IV
       b. II and III
       c. III and IV
       d. I, II, and IV

3. Which particle size is optimal for aerosol deposition in the terminal airways?
   a. >10 μm
   b. 5 to 10 μm
   c. 2 to 5 μm
   d. 0.8 to 3 μm

4. How should a patient be instructed to breathe during an aerosol treatment to achieve optimal drug deposition in the lower respiratory tract?
   a. Slow, deep
   b. Fast, shallow
   c. Slow, shallow
   d. Fast, deep

5. Which aerosol delivery device operates on the piezoelectric principle?
   a. SVNs
   b. SPAGs
   c. DPIs
   d. USNs

6. Advantages of SVNs over other types of delivery devices include all but which of the following?
   a. Little patient coordination required
   b. Is not effective at low inspiratory flows
   c. Inspiratory pause not necessary for efficacy
   d. Is able to aerosolize any drug solution

7. Which of the following aerosol delivery devices requires the patient to be able to generate an inspiratory flow rate of 60 L/min or greater?
   a. USN
   b. SPAG
   c. MDI
   d. DPI

8. Which of the following is true regarding inhalation of a corticosteroid via MDI?
   a. Wait 3 minutes between inhalations.
   b. If a bronchodilator is prescribed, use it after the corticosteroid.
   c. Rinse the mouth and throat with water after inhalation.
   d. It is unnecessary to use a spacer device with a corticosteroid.

9. Which two drugs are currently available in DPI form?
   a. Albuterol and metaproterenol
   b. Salmeterol and albuterol
   c. Cromolyn sodium and isoetharine
   d. Albuterol and cromolyn sodium

10. How much of the total drug dose is delivered to the lung, regardless of the delivery device used?
    a. 10%
    b. 30%
    c. 50%
    d. >50%

11. The size, or MMAD, of aerosol particles that deposit within the nose and mouth is
    a. 10-15 μm
    b. 2-3 μm
    c. 1-2 μm
    d. 20-25 μm

12. For an aerosol to affect the lower lung of a patient with expiratory wheezing you would want to use an SVN that delivered aerosol particle size in the range of:
    a. 10-15 μm
    b. 20-25 μm
    c. 1-5 μm
    d. 0.5-1.0 μm

13. A child is in the ED with croup. The child has severe stridor. When delivering medication to this child your choice of an SVN would be one that delivered a particle size of:
    a. 5-10 μm
    b. 20-25 μm
    c. 1-3 μm
    d. 0.5-1.0 μm

14. With a filling volume of 3-5 ml in an SVN, the flow rate of the nebulizer should be set to:
    a. 4 L/min
    b. 4-5 L/min
    c. 6-10 L/min
    d. >10 L/min

15. When sputtering of the nebulized medication in an SVN occurs, shaking or agitating the SVN will do which of the following to the drug solution delivery?
    a. Increase the volume of drug solution
    b. Decrease the volume of drug solution
    c. Increase the drug solution concentration and delivery of the drug
    d. Have no effect on delivery of the drug solution

16. Which of the following is not a component of an MDI?
    a. Flow rate control
    b. Metering valve
    c. Propellant
    d. Drug

17. To prevent loss of dose when storing a CFC-propelled MDI canister of a drug such as albuterol, you should:
    a. Shake the MDI before storing it
    b. Store the canister in an upright position
    c. Give 2 puffs before storing the canister
    d. Store the canister on its side

18. When instructing a patient in the use of an MDI that delivers corticosteroids, to reduce oropharyngeal impaction of corticosteroids you would tell the patient:
    a. To use an open-mouth technique when inhaling the medication
    b. To use a closed-mouth technique when inhaling the medication
    c. To inhale first and then give the puff of medication
    d. To use a spacer device or holding chamber

19. A patient using an MDI with a spacer device notices a build-up of medication inside the spacer. He is concerned that he is losing medication because it is sticking to the inside of the spacer. To help reduce this loss of medication you would instruct the patient to:
    a. Rinse the inside of the spacer device with vinegar
    b. Rinse the inside of the spacer device with standard household detergent
    c. Exhale into the spacer device before activating the MDI into the spacer
    d. Apply a cloth around the spacer to warm the puff of MDI as it enters the spacer

20. The flow rate needed to disperse the drug of a DPI is:
    a. <30 L/min
    b. 20-40 L/min
    c. 30-90 L/min
    d. >90 L/min

21. Which of the following statements is *true* concerning delivery of a medication during mechanical ventilation of a child or adult?
    a. Using an MDI with a spacer device is better than using an SVN
    b. Using an MDI without a spacer device is better than using an SVN
    c. An SVN is better than an MDI with a spacer device
    d. There is no difference between the use of an SVN and MDI with a spacer device

22. To improve aerosol delivery during mechanical ventilation an SVN should be placed
    a. Directly on the endotracheal tube
    b. Between the Y adapter and the endotracheal tube
    c. 30 cm from the endotracheal tube on the inspiratory side of the patient circuit
    d. Directly behind the heat–moisture exchanger on the inspiratory side of the patient circuit

23. A small volume nebulizer is best for use by which of the following individuals?
    a. A patient able to follow instructions and produce a good breath-hold
    b. A patient with poor inspiratory capacity and who is tachypneic
    c. A patient with stable respiratory drive
    d. A patient with good hand–breath coordination

24. Which of the following aerosol delivery devices could be used for a child 6 months of age and admitted to the ED with a diagnosis of bronchiolitis?
    a. MDI
    b. DPI
    c. SVN
    d. Breath-actuated MDI

25. When administering aerosol agents to a mechanically ventilated patient with a heat–moisture exchanger in place, the respiratory therapist should:
    a. Increase the inspiratory flow rate of the ventilator during the treatment
    b. Bypass the heat–moisture exchanger
    c. Place the aerosol device within 10 cm of the ETT
    d. Only administer the aerosol agent with an SVN

## CASE STUDY

Professor Plum, a 38-year-old male with a history of asthma, presents to the emergency department with a chief complaint of shortness of breath and coughing. His respiratory rate is 34 breaths/min, he is wheezing on both inspiration and expiration throughout both lung fields, and he has accessory muscle usage. He is unable to perform a peak expiratory flow rate maneuver. He complains of anxiety, he is diaphoretic, his heart rate is 148 beats/min, and his oxygen saturation is 92%. He is coughing up thick, white foamy secretions. Oxygen is ordered for Professor Plum by nasal cannula at 2 L/min, as well as aerosol therapy with albuterol.

1. On the basis of this patient's presentation, what would be your recommendation as to the choice of aerosol delivery device?

2. What is your rationale for making this selection?

It is now 48 hours later. The wheezing has subsided considerably, and is now heard slightly on expiration. Professor Plum has a respiratory rate of 18 breaths/min, oxygen saturation is 97% without oxygen, and his heart rate is 96 beats/min. He states that he is not experiencing shortness of breath and in general he is feeling better.

3. On the basis of his physical findings, what would you recommend now?

4. Does he need a reservoir device? Why or why not?

# 4 Calculating Drug Doses

## CHAPTER OBJECTIVES

*After answering the following questions, the reader should be able to:*

1. Use the metric system.
2. Calculate drug doses, using proportions.
3. Calculate drug doses, using percentage-strength solutions.

## KEY TERMS AND DEFINITIONS

*Complete the following questions by writing the answer in the space provided.*

1. The amount of solute in a solution, usually expressed as a percentage, is called the _____.

2. The amount of solute that is in a solution containing 100 parts is the _____.

3. A physically homogeneous mixture of two or more substances is called a(n) _____.

4. A _____ is a substance that is dissolved in a solution.

5. A substance, usually a liquid, that is used to make a solution is called a _____.

6. The amount of drug that is needed, based on a patient's weight, is called _____.

To do drug calculations you've got to use the metric system. (*Hint:* See Table 4-1 in the textbook). Warm up with a few practice conversions:

7. 51 cm = _____ mm

8. 33 g = _____ mg

9. 24 ml = _____ L

10. 17 m = _____ cm

11. 68 kg = _____ grams

Remember that 1 ml = 16 gtts (drops).

12. How many drops in 3 ml? _____

13. How many drops in 0.5 ml? _____

One cubic centimeter (cc) equals 1 ml, so it's best to convert drops to milliliters and draw up medications in a small syringe, such as a tuberculin syringe. All drops are not created equal! The size of the opening and the properties of the liquid can influence the size of the drop.

14. A physician orders 2 drops of a medication. How many milliliters is this? _____

## CALCULATING DOSES FROM PREPARED-STRENGTH LIQUIDS, TABLETS, AND CAPSULES

This section tests your ability to perform three types of calculations: (1) determining drug dose (fluids, tablets, or capsules) based on proportions; (2) calculating drug dose based on percentage-strength solutions; and (3) calculating IV infusion rates.

### Calculating With Proportions

How much liquid, how many tablets, and so on, are needed to provide the right amount of drug to a patient? There are two ways to do this sort of calculation. *Note:* Be sure to convert to consistent units of measure (grams to milliliters, drops to milliliters, etc.)!

Here's where you have a choice: Set up a straightforward proportion:

$$\frac{\text{Original dose}}{\text{Per amount}} = \frac{\text{Desired dose}}{\text{Per amount}}$$

For example: Divalproex is a drug used to treat migraine headaches. It is available in 500-mg tablets. A dosage of 1 g/day is prescribed for a patient. How many tablets should the patient take? First, convert grams to milligrams (1 g = 1000 mg) and list the information for the proportion:

Original dose = 500 mg (amount in 1 tablet)

Per amount = 1 tablet

Desired dose = 1000 mg

Per amount = $x$

So you can do the following (method 1):

$$\frac{500 \text{ mg}}{1 \text{ tablet}} = \frac{1000 \text{ mg}}{x \text{ tablets}}$$

Remember algebra:

$$1000(1) = 500(x)$$

$$1000 = 500(x)$$

$$x = 2 \text{ tablets}$$

15. Drug A comes in 200-mg tablets. A dose of 500 mg/day is prescribed. How many tablets should the patient take?

Let's say the percentage amount changes (just to make it more challenging). My child's cough medicine contains 10 mg of dextromethorphan hydrobromide in 5 ml. If the pediatrician tells me to give 3 ml, how many milligrams have I given?

Original dose = 10 mg

Per amount = 5 ml

Desired dose = x

Per amount = 3 ml

"Plug in" the numbers:

$$\frac{10 \text{ mg}}{5 \text{ ml}} = \frac{x}{3 \text{ ml}}$$
$$10(3) = (x)5$$
$$30 = (x)5$$
$$x = 6 \text{ mg}$$

16. Concerning the same child, you are ordered to give 6 mg of dextromethorphan hydrobromide. How many milliliters of dextromethorphan hydrobromide should be given?

**Drug Amounts in Units**

There are certain drugs, such as insulin and heparin, that come in units instead of milligrams or grams. Set up these types of problems just like the previous ones.

*Example:* Heparin often comes as 1000 U/ml. How many milliliters do you need to give to deliver 650 U of heparin?

Original dose = 1000 units

Per amount = 1 ml

Desired dose = 650 units

Per amount = x ml

$$\frac{1000}{1 \text{ ml}} = \frac{650 \text{ units}}{x \text{ ml}}$$
$$1000(x) = (650)1$$
$$1000(x) = 650$$
$$x = 0.65 \text{ ml}$$

*Note:* Insulin has a standard preparation of 0.04 mg = 1 unit.

## Calculations With a Dosage Schedule

Sometimes it's necessary to calculate drug dosage from a schedule. Remember the term *schedule*? The schedule is the amount of drug needed, based on a person's weight. For example, the average dose of sodium nitroprusside is 3 µg/kg/min. If you have a prepared-strength vial of sodium nitroprusside at 50 µg/ml, how much of that drug preparation should you give to a 70-kg man?

First, calculate the dose you'll need:

$$3 \ \mu g/kg \times 70 \ kg = 210 \ \mu g$$

17. Quick! How many grams is 210 µg? _____

Now calculate the amount of the preparation:

$$\frac{50 \ \mu g}{1 \ ml} = \frac{210 \ \mu g}{x \ ml}$$
$$50(x) = 210$$
$$x = 4.2 \ ml/min$$

## Additional Examples of Calculations With Prepared-Strength Drugs

18. You have terbutaline, 1 mg/ml in an ampoule for injection. How much is needed to give a 0.5-mg dose subcutaneously?

Let's say surfactant is administered at 5 ml/kg. You are asked to determine the dosage for a 1500-g premature infant. First, convert grams to kilograms:

$$1500/1000 = 1.5 \ kg$$

Next, multiply the recommended dose by kilograms:

$$5 \ ml/kg \times 1.5 \ kg = 7.5 \ ml$$

19. A dosage schedule of a surfactant calls for 4 ml/kg of body weight for a 1200-g newborn infant. How many milliliters of surfactant will you need to administer?

## CALCULATING DOSES FROM PERCENTAGE-STRENGTH SOLUTIONS

Keep in mind the definitions at the beginning of this chapter in the workbook.

### Types of Percentage Preparations
Weight to weight: Grams of drug (active ingredient) per 100 g of a mixture
Weight to volume: Grams of drug (active ingredient) per 100 ml of a mixture
Volume to volume: Milliliters of drug (active ingredient) per 100 ml of a mixture

### Solutions by Ratio
When it is necessary to dilute medication for use in aerosol therapy, a solute-to-solvent ratio is often given (e.g., isoproterenol 1:200). A solution of isoproterenol 1:200 means 1 g of isoproterenol per 200 ml of solution. What percent strength is a 1:200 solution of a drug?

$$1 \text{ g}/200 \text{ ml of solution} = 0.005, \text{ which is } 0.5\% \text{ strength } (0.005 \times 100)$$

20. What percent strength is a 1:100 solution of a drug?

Here is another example: albuterol 1:12. This example (ratio by simple parts) indicates actual parts medication to parts solvent. In this case 0.25 ml of albuterol to 3 ml ($0.25 \times 12$) normal saline gives you the 1:12 ratio. *Note:* If the physician had ordered just by the ratio, and you didn't know that 0.25 ml was the usual dose of albuterol, you'd be out of luck.

### Solving Percentage-strength Solution Problems
If the active ingredient is 100% pure and undiluted, use the following equation:

$$\text{Percent strength (in decimals)} = \frac{\text{solute (in grams or cubic centimeters)}}{\text{total amount (solute + solvent)}}$$

For diluted active ingredient use the following equation:

$$\text{Percent strength (in decimals)} = \frac{\text{(dilute solute)} \times \text{(percent strength of solute)}}{\text{total amount (solution)}}$$

Let's do an undiluted active ingredient problem: How many milligrams of active ingredient are there in 5 ml of a 1:500 drug that prevents belching?

First, figure out the percentage strength. Always do this first!

$$\text{Percent strength is } 1:500 = 0.002$$

$$\text{Total amount of solution} = 5 \text{ ml}$$

$$\text{Active ingredient} = x \text{ ml}$$

$$0.002 = x \text{ g}/5 \text{ ml}$$

$$x \text{ g} = 0.002 \times 5 = 0.01 \text{ g of active ingredient}$$

21. But wait. The question asked how many milligrams, so don't forget to convert! The answer is _____ mg.

22. How many milligrams of active ingredient are there in 5 ml of a 1:250 drug?

Now for an example requiring the diluted active ingredient equation: How much 10% Mucomyst is needed to prepare 3 ml of 20% Mucomyst? (10% and 20% indicate that the Mucomyst is not 100% pure. That's why the equation for diluted active ingredient is needed).

$$\text{Percent strength (in decimals)} = 0.20$$

$$\text{Total amount of solution} = 3 \text{ ml}$$

$$\text{Active ingredient percent strength} = 0.10$$

$$\text{Dilute solute (active ingredient)} = x \text{ ml}$$

$$0.20 = x(0.10)/3 \text{ ml}$$

$$x(0.10) = 0.20 \times 3$$

$$x(0.10) = 0.6$$

$$x = 0.6/0.10 = 6 \text{ cc of 10% Mucomyst (Bring a good book,}$$
$$\text{as this treatment will last forever!)}$$

23. A patient needs 3 cc of 10% Mucomyst, but only 20% Mucomyst is available. How much 20% Mucomyst should be used?

### Some Do's and Don'ts

- Do give your answer in the units that are asked for in the question!
- Don't forget to use decimals when solving percent strength problems!
- Do convert to metric units!

24. Which of the following doses is more dilute: 5 mg of active ingredient in 3 ml, or 5 mg of active ingredient in 6 ml?

## NATIONAL BOARD FOR RESPIRATORY CARE–TYPE QUESTIONS

Here are 10 examples of NBRC calculations.

1. The respiratory care practitioner (RCP) is asked to add 1 g of metaproterenol to 100 ml of aqueous solvent. This will result in which of the following concentrations?
    I. 1:1000
    II. 0.01
    III. 1:100
    IV. 1%
        a. I and II
        b. II and III
        c. III and IV
        d. I and IV

2. You are asked to administer 1 ml of a 1% solution of isoetharine to an asthmatic patient. How many milligrams of drug is this?
    a. 1 mg
    b. 10 mg
    c. 100 mg
    d. 1000 mg

3. The physician's order reads, "Administer 5 mg of metaproterenol via SVN." How many milliliters of a 1:100 solution should be used?
    a. 0.5
    b. 1
    c. 1.5
    d. 2

4. The RCP is asked to dilute 100 ml of a 2% solution of beclomethasone to a 1% solution. How many milliliters of water must be added to the original mixture to produce the desired concentration?
    a. 100
    b. 50
    c. 200
    d. 150

5. How many milliliters of water are needed to dilute 10 ml of a 20% solution of acetylcysteine to a 5% concentration?
    a. 40
    b. 60
    c. 50
    d. 20

6. The physician's order reads, "Instill 5 ml 5% NaHCO$_3$ q4h and prn." The pharmacy has 50-ml ampoules of an 8.4% solution. How many milliliters of distilled water must be added to make a 5% solution?
   a. 10
   b. 21
   c. 34
   d. 42

7. The physician's order reads, "Administer 75 mg decadron via hand-held nebulizer." How many milliliters of a 2.5% solution should you use?
   a. 2.2
   b. 0.5
   c. 3
   d. 1.5

8. You need to administer 1 L of normal saline to a patient at a drip rate of 15 drops/min. The standard drop factor of the IV set is 15 drops/ml. How long will it take to deliver it?
   a. 250 minutes
   b. 500 minutes
   c. 1000 minutes
   d. 1500 minutes

9. What is the percent strength of a drug available at 50 mg/ml?
   a. 1
   b. 5
   c. 10
   d. 15

10. The usual dosage of albuterol sulfate is 0.5 ml of a 0.5% strength solution. How many milligrams is this?
    a. 5.0
    b. 2.5
    c. 1.25
    d. 0.50

## CASE STUDY 1

A resident orders cromolyn sodium to be delivered via SVN to one of your patients. The drug is available as 20 mg in 2 ml of aqueous solution. What percentage strength are you delivering to your patient? (*Hint:* You're doing a weight-to-volume calculation.)

A 45-year-old patient is admitted to the intensive care unit with Tylenol overdose. The treatment calls for administration of 6 ml of 20% Mucomyst. Only 10% Mucomyst is available. How much 10% Mucomyst is needed to prepare 6 ml of 20% Mucomyst?

# 5 The Central and Peripheral Nervous Systems

## CHAPTER OBJECTIVES

*After answering the following questions, the reader should be able to:*

1. Classify the branches of the nervous system
2. Differentiate between the *central, peripheral*, and *autonomic nervous systems*
3. Discuss the use of *neurotransmitters*
4. Explain in detail the difference between the *parasympathetic* and *sympathetic* branches of the nervous system
5. Differentiate the effects of *cholinergic* and *anticholinergic agents* on the nervous system
6. Differentiate the effects of *adrenergic* and *antiadrenergic agents* on the nervous system
7. Discuss the various receptors in the airways
8. Differentiate between *nonadrenergic, noncholinergic inhibitory*, and *excitatory* nerves

## KEY TERMS AND DEFINITIONS

*Complete the following questions by writing the correct term in the blank provided.*

1. The part of the nervous system that includes the brain and spinal cord, controlling voluntary and involuntary acts,

    is called the _____ _____ _____.

2. The portion of the nervous system that is outside the central nervous system and includes the sensory, sympa-

    thetic, and parasympathetic nerves is known as the _____ _____

    _____.

3. Signals that are transmitted from the brain and spinal cord are called _____.

4. Signals that are transmitted to the brain and spinal cord are called _____.

5. The neurotransmitter used at most sympathetic nerve sites is _____.

6. A chemical produced by the body and that is used in the transmission of nerve impulses is

    _____. It is destroyed by cholinesterase.

7. A drug stimulating a receptor for norepinephrine or epinephrine is called _____.

8. A drug blocking a receptor for acetylcholine is called _____.

9. An agent causing stimulation of parasympathetic nervous system sites is called _____.

10. An agent that blocks the effect of the sympathetic nervous system is called _____.

11. An agent that blocks the effect of the parasympathetic nervous system is called _____.

12. An agent that stimulates the sympathetic nervous system is called _____.

*Complete the following questions by writing the correct term in the blank provided.*

13. In your body there are two major control systems: these include the _____ system and the

    _____ system.

14. The nervous system is divided into three parts. Name each part.

    a. _____

    b. _____

    c. _____

15. The parasympathetic and sympathetic nervous systems are contained in the _____ nervous
    system.

16. Because sympathetic fibers innervate the adrenal medulla, when sympathetic activation occurs there is a release of

    _____ into the blood stream.

17. The parasympathetic branch arises from the _____ portion of the spinal cord.

18. The sympathetic branch arises from the _____ portion of the spinal cord.

Figure 5-1 in the textbook gives you an overview of the central and peripheral nervous systems, including the autonomic
branches (sympathetic and parasympathetic).

19. List three characteristics of the parasympathetic nervous system and three characteristics of the sympathetic nervous
    system.

    **Parasympathetic nervous system**

    a. _____

    b. _____

    c. _____

    **Sympathetic nervous system**

    a. _____

    b. _____

    c. _____

20. Give one example of when you'd want your sympathetic nervous system to be activated.




Figure 5-1 in the textbook also summarizes the usual neurotransmitters in the peripheral nervous system. *Note:* To understand autonomic drugs, you need to understand neurotransmitters.

21. Neurotransmitters control _____ impulses.

22. The neurotransmitter *everywhere* (skeletal muscle, parasympathetic nervous system terminal nerve sites, and all

    ganglionic synapses), except at sympathetic terminal nerve sites, is _____.

23. Circle the correct answer: The autonomic nervous system is generally thought to be an (efferent/afferent) system.

24. The neurotransmitter conducting the nerve impulse at skeletal muscle sites is _____.

25. Sympathetic fibers that have acetylcholine at the neuroeffector site are _____.

26. Match each of the following terms with its corresponding definition below.

    1. _____ Sympathomimetic
    
    2. _____ Adrenergic
    
    3. _____ Parasympatholytic
    
    4. _____ Anticholinergic
    
    5. _____ Antiadrenergic
    
    6. _____ Parasympathomimetic
    
    7. _____ Cholinergic
    
    8. _____ Sympatholytic

    a. Agent blocking sympathetic nervous system
    b. Agent stimulating parasympathetic nervous system
    c. Agent blocking epinephrine receptor
    d. Agent blocking acetylcholine receptor
    e. Agent stimulating sympathetic nervous system
    f. Agent stimulating acetylcholine receptor
    g. Agent blocking parasympathetic nervous system
    h. Agent stimulating epinephrine receptor

## Parasympathetic Branch

The lung is supplied by vagus nerves that innervate the trachea. Branches of the vagus nerves innervate the hilum and smaller airways. The vagus nerves release acetylcholine and are therefore termed *cholinergic*. When acetylcholine combines with certain receptors (muscarinic) on airway smooth muscle, bronchoconstriction occurs. When acetylcholine combines with receptors on submucosal glands, more mucus is produced. Acetylcholine is kept at the proper levels by an enzyme called cholinesterase, which breaks down acetylcholine.

27. In the following, fill in the changes that occur with parasympathetic stimulation:

    a. Heart: _____ _____

    b. Bronchial smooth muscle: _____

    c. Exocrine glands: _____ _____

28. Two additional terms used to refer to stimulation of receptor sites by acetylcholine are

_____, because of the effect of nicotine, and _____, because of the effect of muscarine.

29. Circle the correct answer: Administration of a muscarinic drug such as neostigmine will (increase/decrease) airway secretions.

30. A parasympathomimetic effect is the same as a _____ effect, and a parasympatholytic

effect is the same as a _____ effect.

## CHOLINERGIC AND ANTICHOLINERGIC AGENTS

*Complete the following questions by writing the answer in the space provided.*

31. Name a direct-acting cholinergic drug that is used to assess the degree of airway reactivity in

asthmatics: _____

32. Drugs such as parasympatholytics and neuromuscular blocking agents block acetylcholine receptors and therefore

are called _____ agents.

33. An antihistamine drug with an anticholinergic effect, commonly used to prevent motion sickness,

is _____.

34. Give four uses of a parasympatholytic or antimuscarinic agent such as atropine.

a. _____

b. _____

c. _____

d. _____

35. Circle the correct answer: Stimulation of the heart will (increase/decrease) cardiac output.

36. The neurotransmitter at the terminal nerve sites in the sympathetic branch of the autonomic nervous

system is _____.

37. The following are sympathomimetic drugs. Fill in their uses.

| Drug | Uses |
|------|------|
| Epinephrine | a. _____ |
| Albuterol | b. _____ |
| Salmeterol | c. _____ |
| Dopamine | d. _____ |

38. What are two types of sympathetic receptors?

    a. _____

    b. _____

39. Stimulation of alpha (α) receptors causes _____.

40. Stimulation of beta$_1$ (β$_1$) receptors increases the _____ and _____

    _____ _____ of cardiac smooth muscle.

41. Stimulation of β$_2$ receptors causes _____ and _____ muscle relaxation.

42. Which receptors (α, β$_1$, or β$_2$) would be best to stimulate if the patient had a runny nose?

43. Which receptors (α, β$_1$, or β$_2$) would be best to stimulate to give relief to a patient in the midst of an asthma attack?

So in general, α$_1$ and β$_1$ receptors excite, and α$_2$ and β$_2$ receptors inhibit.

44. A drug such as propranolol, an antiarryhthmic, blocks the sympathetic adrenergic effects. Because of these effects

    it would be categorized as a _____.

## NEURAL CONTROL OF LUNG FUNCTION

Both the parasympathetic and sympathetic branches of the autonomic nervous system control lung function to some extent.

*Complete the following questions by writing the correct term in the blank provided.*

45. Although there's no direct sympathetic innervation of airway smooth muscle, the sympathetic nervous system

    controls smooth muscle tone by circulating _____ and _____.

46. Epinephrine will act on both _____ and _____ receptors whereas

    norepinephrine acts primarily on _____ receptors.

47. β Agonists, distributed from the trachea to terminal bronchioles, cause _____ of small airways.

48. True or False: Adrenergic receptors in the lung are all β$_2$ receptors.

49. True or False: β$_1$ Receptors are located in the alveolar walls and lung periphery.

50. True or False: The α receptors are located equally throughout large and small airways and are less in quantity than β receptors.

51. The lung receives its blood supply from both the _____ and the

   _____ circulations.

52. Pulmonary circulation is innervated by both the _____ _____

   _____ and the _____ _____

   _____.

53. Arterial (bronchial) circulation is innervated mostly by the _____

   _____ _____.

54. Bronchial submucosal glands are innervated by the _____ _____

   _____ and _____ _____

   _____.

55. Submucosal glands have both _____ and _____ receptors.

56. The lung is innervated by the _____ nerve, which enters the lung at the hilum and innervates intrapulmonary airways.

57. Stimulation of the vagus nerve causes _____.

58. Circle the correct answer: Stimulation of the vagus nerve also causes submucosal glands to (increase/decrease) secretions.

59. There are three muscarinic receptor sites in the lung. Which of these, $M_1$, $M_2$, or $M_3$, is located on submucosal

   glands and airway smooth muscle? _____

60. Muscarinic receptor M3 is located on blood vessels, causing the release of endothelial-derived relaxant factor

   producing _____ of the both bronchial and pulmonary vasculature.

## NATIONAL BOARD FOR RESPIRATORY CARE–TYPE QUESTIONS

*Now that you've had a chance to review this material from the text, try answering the following questions. When you're finished, check your responses with the answer key at the end of the book.*

1. The sympathetic nervous system is part of which of the following?
   a. Central nervous system
   b. Peripheral nervous system
   c. Autonomic nervous system
   d. Both b and c

2. Which branch of the nervous system controls daily functions such as digestion and bladder control?
   a. Central nervous system
   b. Parasympathetic nervous system
   c. Sympathetic nervous system
   d. Both b and c

3. Which of the following describes a drug that stimulates the sympathetic nervous system?
   a. Parasympathomimetic
   b. Parasympatholytic
   c. Sympathomimetic
   d. Sympatholytic

4. Which of the following describes the autonomic nervous system?
   a. Sends impulses from the brain to the neuroeffector sites (e.g., heart and lungs)
   b. Sends impulses from the periphery to the brain and spinal cord
   c. Is exemplified by the knee-jerk reaction
   d. Is an afferent system

5. Which of the following describes a drug that blocks a receptor for acetylcholine?
   a. Cholinergic
   b. Anticholinergic
   c. Adrenergic
   d. Antiadrenergic

6. Sympathetic nervous system stimulation results in all but which of the following?
   a. Increased blood pressure
   b. Mental stimulation
   c. Increased urine output
   d. Bronchodilation

7. Which two enzymes inactivate catecholamines?
   a. TDH and BHG
   b. COTN and MNM
   c. DDT and TKO
   d. COMT and MAO

8. Stimulation of which of the following receptors results in vasoconstriction?
   a. $\alpha$
   b. $\beta_1$
   c. $\beta_2$
   d. $\gamma$

9. Epinephrine accomplishes which of the following?
   a. Stimulates primarily $\alpha$ receptors
   b. Stimulates primarily $\beta$ receptors
   c. Stimulates $\alpha$ and $\beta$ receptors equally
   d. Stimulates neither $\alpha$ nor $\beta$ receptors

10. Blood flow to the lung is supplied by which of the following?
    I. Pulmonary circulation
    II. Vagal circulation
    III. Bronchial circulation
    IV. Parasympathetic circulation
       a. I and IV only
       b. II and III only
       c. I and III only
       d. II and IV only

11. Bronchodilation most likely occurs because of stimulation of which receptor?
    a. $\alpha_1$
    b. $\alpha_2$
    c. $\beta_1$
    d. $\beta_2$

12. Relaxation of airway smooth muscle should *not* occur with which of the following?
    a. Stimulation of the nonadrenergic inhibitory nerves
    b. Use of a cholinergic agent
    c. Use of a sympathomimetic
    d. Use of a parasympatholytic

13. A drug that stimulates the parasympathetic nervous system will cause which of the following?
    a. Slower heart rate
    b. Bronchodilation
    c. Reduced secretions
    d. Thicker secretions

14. Which of the following is *not* a sympathomimetic or adrenergic agonist?
    a. Epinephrine
    b. Propranolol
    c. Albuterol
    d. Salmeterol

15. Adrenergic receptors in the lung are:
    a. All $\alpha_1$
    b. All $\beta_1$
    c. All $\beta_2$
    d. $\alpha_1$ and $\beta_2$

16. Bronchial submucosal glands are innervated by:
    a. Parasympathetic nervous system
    b. Sympathetic nervous system
    c. Both parasympathetic and sympathetic nervous systems
    d. Central nervous system

17. The nerve that innervates the lung and enters at the hilum is the:
    a. Phrenic
    b. Pulmonic
    c. Glossopharyngeal
    d. Vagus

18. Stimulation of $\beta_1$ receptors of cardiac smooth muscle will cause which of the following?
    I. Increased heart rate
    II. Reduced cardiac output
    III. Coronary artery constriction
    IV. Increased force of contraction
        a. I and III only
        b. I and IV only
        c. I, II, and III only
        d. I, II, III, and IV

19. Which of the following agonists would be best for a patient to give relief in the midst of an asthma attack?
    a. $\alpha_1$
    b. $\beta_1$
    c. $\alpha_2$
    d. $\beta_2$

20. Which of the following would *not* be a sympathomimetic effect of epinephrine?
    a. Bronchodilation
    b. Antiarryhthmic
    c. Vasoconstriction
    d. Cardiac stimulation

## CASE STUDY 1

Methacholine is an inhaled parasympathomimetic agent used in bronchial challenge tests to determine the degree of airway reactivity in asthmatic individuals.

1. What is the parasympathetic effect?

2. How might methacholine work to detect the degree of airway reactivity?

# 6 Adrenergic (Sympathomimetic) Bronchodilators

## CHAPTER OBJECTIVES

*After answering the following questions the reader should be able to:*

1. Define *sympathomimetic*
2. Define *adrenergic*
3. List all currently available β-adrenergic agents used in respiratory therapy
4. Differentiate between the specific adrenergic agents and formulations
5. Describe the mode of action for each specific adrenergic agent and formulation
6. Describe the route of administration available for β agonists
7. Discuss adverse effects of β agonists
8. Clinically assess β-agonist therapy

## KEY TERMS AND DEFINITIONS

*Complete the following questions by writing the correct answer in the blank provided.*

1. An enzyme that produces a reaction the opposite of that of cAMP, and causes bronchoconstriction,

   is _____.

2. A _____ produces effects similar to those of the sympathetic nervous system.

3. Narrowing of the airways due to contraction of smooth muscle is called _____.

4. A group of similar compounds having sympathomimetic action and mimicking the actions of epinephrine

   are the _____.

5. An agent that stimulates sympathetic nervous fibers and allows relaxation of smooth muscle in the airway is a(n)

   _____ _____.

6. A drug that exhibits pharmacological activity once it is converted, inside the body, to its active form, is called a

   _____.

7. _____ _____ causes vasoconstriction and a vasopressor effect in the upper airway, which provides decongestion.

8. _____ _____ causes increase myocardial conductivity and increased heart rate as well as increased contractile force.

9. Long-term desensitization of β receptors to $\beta_2$ agonists, caused by a reduction in the number of β receptors, is

   called _____.

10. _____ _____ causes relaxation of bronchial smooth muscle with some inhibition of inflammatory mediator release and stimulation of mucociliary clearance.

Chapter 6 is of particular importance, because inhaled adrenergic bronchodilators represent the drugs most commonly administered by respiratory care practitioners.

Adrenergic drugs work by stimulating $\beta_2$ receptors on bronchial smooth muscle. Some adrenergic drugs (at or near the top of Table 6-1 in the textbook) also stimulate $\alpha$ and $\beta_1$ receptors.

11. What are the results of $\alpha$ and $\beta_1$ stimulation?

Vasoconstriction, decongestion, and increased heart rate and force of contraction are not what we want! $\beta_2$-Specific drugs produce the following:

■ Relaxation of bronchial smooth muscle
■ Inhibition of inflammatory mediator release
■ Stimulation of mucociliary clearance

The clear trend in pharmaceutical development is toward agents that are more $\beta_2$ specific (with few $\beta_1$-specific effects).

*Circle either* heart *or* lung *in the next sentence.*

12. "$\beta_2$ Specific" means more of the desired effect on the (heart, lung) and less effect on the (heart, lung).

## CLINICAL INDICATION FOR ADRENERGIC BRONCHODILATORS

13. What is the general indication for adrenergic bronchodilators?

14. What are three examples of short-acting adrenergic bronchodilators?

15. Short-acting adrenergic bronchodilators are useful for relaxation of airway smooth muscle in the presence of

reversible airflow obstruction associated with _____.

16. List three long-acting adrenergic bronchodilators.

17. These long-acting adrenergic bronchodilators are useful for

    a. Control of _____

    b. Control of _____ symptoms of asthma

18. Short-acting adrenergic bronchodilators are termed _____ whereas long-acting adrenergic

    bronchodilators are termed _____.

## Catecholamines

The following are words to live by: All sympathomimetic bronchodilators are catecholamines or derivatives of catecholamines. A *catecholamine* is a sympathomimetic amine, and it mimicks the action of epinephrine.

19. List three examples of catecholamines (and you already have one of these).

20. Put a check mark next to the symptom(s) that occur(s) with administration of a catecholamine:

    a. Tachycardia: _____

    b. Bronchoconstriction: _____

    c. Elevated blood pressure: _____

    d. Bronchodilation: _____

    e. Increased urine output: _____

    f. Relaxation of skeletal muscle blood vessels: _____

Now let's learn more about the drugs, beginning with epinephrine.

21. Epinephrine is a potent catecholamine bronchodilator, but it also gives you _____ and

    _____ stimulation.

22. Epinephrine can administered by _____ and _____.

23. Why can't catecholamines be given orally?

Remember that epinephrine works quickly (rapid onset) but doesn't last long because it is metabolized by catechol *O*-methyltransferase (COMT), a cytoplasmic enzyme found in the liver, kidneys, and other parts of the body.

You might hear of a drug called racemic epinephrine, which is a synthetic form of epinephrine. It also gives both α and β effects, but with about half the vasoconstrictor effect. It's great for topical administration or inhalation, and is sometimes used to treat croup.

24. If racemic epinephrine is being nebulized for croup, should the respiratory therapist instruct the patient to take deep breaths with intermittent breath-holding? Why?

How were the catecholamines made more $\beta_2$ specific? It's basically explained by the keyhole theory of β sympathomimetic receptors. Catecholamines have a catechol base and an amine side chain (analogous to a key). The longer and more complex the side chain, the more $\beta_2$ specific the drug.

Don't forget that a limitation of all these drugs is that they are inactivated by COMT, found mainly in the liver and gut. The effects of all the drugs we've talked about so far last only 1 to 3 hours.

Resorcinol agents were created by modifying the catechol nucleus, so that it would no longer be inactivated by COMT. What a triumph!

25. Among the resorcinol agents are metaproterenol and terbutaline (although available only for IV administration). These are better than the unmodified catecholamines because they do which of the following [check the correct one(s)]?

a. Last longer (up to 6 hours): _____

b. Are $\beta_2$ specific, with minimal cardiac side effects: _____

c. Cannot be taken orally (not vulnerable to COMT): _____

d. Are slower to peak, which makes them a better choice for maintenance therapy: _____

e. Quick onset, more potent bronchodilators: _____

f. Better for maintenance therapy: _____

**Saligenins**
Saligenins resulted from a different modification of the catechol nucleus. An example is albuterol.

26. List three ways in which albuterol can be delivered.

27. List the advantages of albuterol.

## Pirbuterol (Maxair)

Pirbuterol (Maxair) is also a noncatecholamine adrenergic drug. It is available only for metered dose inhaler (MDI) administration with a breath-actuated inhaler delivery device.

28. Check all of the following that apply to Pirbuterol (Maxair):

    a. Onset of action is 5-8 minutes: _____

    b. Peak effect occurs at about 30 minutes, lasts about 5 hours: _____

    c. Usual dose is 2 puffs: _____

    d. Strength per puff is 0.2 mg: _____

    e. It comes in tablets: _____

    f. It is a catecholamine adrenergic agent: _____

## Bitolterol: (Tornalate)

Bitolterol is called a *prodrug*.

29. What is a prodrug?

Imagine that bitolterol is administered as an inhalation solution. It's gradually hydrolyzed by esterase enzymes, releasing colterol (the active drug). *Voilà!*

30. Bitolterol has a sustained release effect (like the cold capsules on TV ads), and it lasts about

    _____.

## Levalbuterol (Xopenex): The (R)-isomer of Albuterol

31. Nebulized solutions of levalbuterol are available in three strengths. What are they?

32. Levalbuterol is now available in what form of MDI?

33. Check all of the following that apply to levalbuterol (Xopenex):

   a. Duration is 5-8 hours: _____

   b. Onset of action is 15 minutes: _____

   c. Peak effect is 30-60 minutes: _____

   d. It is now available in syrup: _____

   e. It is available as a dry powder inhaler (DPI): _____

## Long-Acting β-Adrenergic Agents

The drugs that we've discussed so far share the limitation of lasting up to 8 hours. This presents a problem for patients who need overnight control of nocturnal symptoms of asthma. It's also easier for patients to take a pill or MDI two times a day than four times a day, so this category of drugs might lead to better compliance.

   Examples of these drugs include salmeterol (Serevent), formoterol (Foradil), and extended-release or sustained-release albuterol.

34. For the drugs salmeterol, formoterol, and arformoterol, which of the following is true? (review Table 6-1).

   a. Available as a small volume nebulizer (SVN): _____

   b. Available as a DPI: _____

   c. Duration is up to 12 hours: _____

   d. Peak effect is 3-5 hours: _____

   e. Has $\beta_2$ effects: _____

   f. Peak effect is 30-60 minutes: _____

Sustained release albuterol is available as Proventil Repetabs or Volmax. Repetabs are pills that contain half the dose in the coating (for immediate release) and half in the core (for release after several hours).

35. Proventil Repetabs or Volmax Repetabs has a duration of activity of up to _____.

Salmeterol also inhibits histamine for up to 20 hours—a definite plus. But don't use it as a substitute for corticosteroids.
   The important thing to remember about the long-acting adrenergic drugs: Do not use them to treat an acute asthma attack!

36. Salmeterol is a _____-_____ receptor agonist and is available in a

   _____ _____ formulation in the Diskus Inhaler.

37. Why is it a bad idea to use long-lasting adrenergic drugs during an acute asthma attack?

Salmeterol is used by patients who have asthma, need to use a β agonist every day, and need to use inhaled corticosteroids or prophylactic agents to keep their asthma under control.

38. The time to peak bronchodilating effect of salmeterol is _____ hours and its duration of action in maintaining the forced expiratory volume in 1 second ($FEV_1$) above pretreatment baseline is

    _____ hours.

39. The U.S. Food and Drug Administration (FDA) approved formoterol for the treatment of asthma for which group of patients?

40. Which group of patients would benefit from the use of formoterol for prevention of acute exercise-induced bronchospasm?

41. Formoterol (Foradil) is a $β_2$-selective agonist with a bronchodilating effect for up to _____ hours,

    with the onset of bronchodilation occurring within a range of _____ minutes.

42. Besides long-acting bronchodilation, what other effect does formoterol have that helps reduce airway resistance?

43. Circle True or False in the following statements:

    a. True or False: National guidelines recommend the introduction of salmeterol in asthma requiring step 3 care.

    b. True or False: Use of long-acting β agonists may prevent the need to increase the inhaled dose of corticosteroid.

    c. True or False: Long-acting $β_2$ agonists are recommended for rescue bronchodilation.

d. True or False: Asthmatics must be educated in the use of both short-acting and long-acting bronchodilators.

e. True or False: Both the short-acting and long-acting $\beta_2$ agonists can be substituted for inhaled corticosteroids because of their antiinflammatory effects.

f. True or False: When discussing the rate of onset of bronchodilating effects, salmeterol can be classified as slow and formoterol as fast.

g. True or False: The Advair Diskus inhaler is a combination product of both salmeterol and fluticasone that has demonstrated superior asthma control and better lung function than either drug taken alone.

44. Symbicort, administered by MDI, is a combination of budesonide and formoterol and is approved for the treatment of asthma in patients _____ years of age and older.

## MODE OF ACTION

45. Match the following modes of action with the type of receptor stimulation:

a. _____ Upper airway vasoconstriction

b. _____ Relaxation of bronchial smooth muscle

c. _____ Stimulation of mucociliary clearance

d. _____ Increased heart rate

e. _____ Decongestion in the nasal passages

f. _____ Increased contractile force of the heart

g. _____ Some inhibition of inflammatory mediator release

1. $\alpha$-Receptor stimulation
2. $\beta_1$-Receptor stimulation
3. $\beta_2$-Receptor stimulation

## ROUTES OF ADMINISTRATION

46. The following is a list of routes of administration. Indicate for each route whether it is currently available (Y for Yes) or not available (N for No) for $\beta$-adrenergic bronchodilators:

a. MDI: _____

b. DPI: _____

c. Tablet: _____

d. Syrup: _____

e. Nebulizer solution: _____

f. Parenteral: _____

g. Suppository: _____

47. List five reasons why inhalation is the preferred route of administration of a β-adrenergic drug:

   a. _____

   b. _____

   c. _____

   d. _____

   e. _____

48. What group of drugs must be given by inhalation because they are ineffective orally?

49. A practical approach to optimal drug dosing in a patient brought to the emergency department with severe airway obstruction, and who does not respond to intermittent nebulizer treatments after an hour, would be

   _____ _____ of β agonists, using a large-reservoir nebulizer such as the Heart nebulizer.

50. What are five advantages of the oral route in administering β agonists?

   a. _____

   b. _____

   c. _____

   d. _____

   e. _____

## ADVERSE SIDE EFFECTS

In general, the term *side effect* denotes any effect other than the desired therapeutic effect. The most common side effects of (*S*)-albuterol are listed in Box 6-1 in the textbook. The more recently developed bronchodilators, being more $\beta_2$ specific, are less likely to cause many of the side effects seen with the earlier bronchodilators (the catecholamines). Stimulation of $\beta_2$ receptors in skeletal muscle may cause muscle tremors. Peripheral vasodilation may cause a reflex tachycardia. It is possible that $\beta_2$ receptors also are present on heart muscle, and stimulation may result in an increased heart rate.

51. What does the term *side effect* indicate?

Reduced effectiveness of a drug with use over time, referred to as *tolerance*, is a concern. *In vitro* studies show both acute and chronic desensitization with bronchodilator use. In the clinical setting, the use of inhaled β agonists does result in a decreased peak effect, but the bronchodilator response remains significant and stabilizes within several weeks with continued use. Diminished side effects, such as tremors, are a result of regular use of inhaled β-agonist bronchodilators. Inflammation also may desensitize receptors. Corticosteroids can reverse the desensitization of β receptors.

52. What does tolerance mean?

There is a difference between bronchodilation and the bronchoprotective effect of β agonists. The bronchodilating effect can be measured on the basis of airflow changes such as $FEV_1$ and peak expiratory flow rate (PEFR). The bronchoprotective effect refers to the reaction of the airways to provocative stimuli such as allergens or irritants and is measured with doses of histamine, methacholine, or cold air. Studies have found that the protective effect of bronchodilators declines more rapidly than that of the bronchodilating effect and that tolerance occurs with the protective effect just as it does with bronchodilation.

53. Bronchodilating effects can be measured on the basis of _____

_____ such as $FEV_1$ or PEFR. Bronchoprotective effects can be measured by

administration of _____, _____, or _____

_____.

Side effects caused by CNS stimulation by adrenergic bronchodilators include headache, nervousness, irritability, anxiety, insomnia, dizziness, and nausea.

A fall in arterial oxygen pressure ($PaO_2$) during bronchodilator administration has been noted. The mechanism seems to be the result of ventilation–perfusion mismatching, with increased perfusion in poorly ventilated areas of the lung. Routinely the drop in $PaO_2$ is physiologically negligible, with drops rarely exceeding a 10-mmHg change. Oxygen tensions usually return to baseline within 30 minutes.

Adrenergic bronchodilators can increase blood glucose and insulin levels and cause a decrease in potassium levels. This is a normal effect of sympathomimetics. These metabolic effects are minimal with inhaled β-adrenergic agents because plasma levels of the drug remain low.

Use of the Freon-powered MDIs can cause bronchospasm in hyperreactive airways. This was found to occur in a small number of individuals (4%) and lasted only a short time (<3 minutes).

There are no noticeable differences in adverse reactions among patients using a CFC MDI and those using an HFA MDI. DPIs, SVNs, and oral medication are alternative routes if this side effect is severe.

54. A fall in $PaO_2$ during bronchodilator delivery seems to be the result of

_____–_____ mismatching.

Hyperreactive airways sensitive to sulfite preservatives will develop bronchospasm. Most commonly used bronchodilators no longer use sulfites as preservatives. It is recommended that only additive-free, sterile-filled unit dose bronchodilator solutions be used for acute airflow obstruction. If side effects of coughing and wheezing are encountered after aerosol treatments, additives and preservatives should be investigated as a possible cause.

## β-AGONIST CONTROVERSY

Despite our increased understanding of asthma and the availability of improved drug treatment, asthma morbidity and mortality seem to be increasing. The *asthma paradox* is a term used to describe this phenomenon. The role that $β_2$ drugs play in this phenomenon is unclear. On the basis of a review of the literature, the following conclusions are presented:
- Use of β agonists may allow allergic individuals to expose themselves to allergens and stimuli leading to increased bronchial hyperresponsiveness
- Repeated self-administration of β agonists may lead to underestimation of the severity of asthma symptoms

- Use of β agonists to alleviate symptoms of wheezing and resistance may lead to insufficient use of antiinflammatory agents
- There is increased airway irritation with environment pollutants and lifestyle changes
- Accumulation of the (S)-isomer with racemic β agonists could exert a detrimental effect on asthma control

## RESPIRATORY CARE ASSESSMENT OF β-AGONIST THERAPY

55. Circle True or False in the following statements:
    a. True or False: A peak flow meter can be used to assess the reversibility of airflow obstruction at the bedside.

    b. True or False: The respiratory care practitioner should assess breathing rate and pattern and breath sounds before and after the completion of treatment.

    c. True or False: Potassium can decrease and blood glucose can increase with the use of continuous nebulization.

    d. True or False: When educating a patient about asthma it should be emphasized that only β agonists are needed to prevent severe asthma episodes.

    e. True or False: Patient education should include the correct use of aerosol devices as well as assembly and cleaning of devices.

    f. True or False: When assessing a patient to determine the benefit of long-acting β agonists, the respiratory care practitioner should assess nocturnal symptoms, number of exacerbations, unscheduled clinic or hospital visits, and days of absence from work due to symptoms.

## NATIONAL BOARD OF RESPIRATORY CARE–TYPE QUESTIONS

1. $β_2$-Receptor stimulation can have all but which of the following effects?
   a. Mucous gland hypertrophy
   b. Bronchial smooth muscle relaxation
   c. Inhibition of histamine release
   d. Stimulation of mucociliary clearance

2. Catecholamines do which of the following?
   a. Mimic the action of catechol
   b. Mimic the action of epinephrine
   c. Have a prolamine nucleus
   d. Are α inhibitors

3. Which of the following describes catecholamines?
   a. Long-acting
   b. Slow onset
   c. Useful for asthma maintenance therapy
   d. Inactivated by COMT

4. Catecholamines are unsuitable for which route of administration?
   a. IV
   b. Inhalation
   c. Oral
   d. Subcutaneous

5. Metaproterenol is an example of which type of adrenergic bronchodilator?
   a. Catecholamine
   b. Resorcinol
   c. Saligenin
   d. Sustained release

6. Which of the following statements are true of bitolterol?
    I. It is converted to colterol in the body.
    II. It is administered by tablet.
    III. Colterol is a catecholamine.
    IV. Its effects can last up to 8 hours.
        a. I, II, III, and IV
        b. I, II, and III only
        c. I, III, and IV only
        d. I, III, and IV only

7. All but which of the following are side effects associated with the use of adrenergic bronchodilators?
        a. Worsening ventilation–perfusion
        b. Hypotension
        c. Nausea
        d. Tachycardia

8. Your patient is receiving metaproterenol 0.25 ml in 3 ml of normal saline. Her heart rate increases from 80 to 120 beats/min. She complains of tremor and palpitations. What should you recommend to her physician?
        a. Initiate continuous nebulization
        b. Decrease the dose
        c. Switch to a drug with greater $\beta_2$ specificity
        d. Either b or c

9. Which of the following catecholamines or catecholamine derivatives lasts the longest?
        a. Isoproterenol
        b. Terbutaline
        c. Metaproterenol
        d. Salmeterol

10. All but which of the following diseases is likely to respond well to adrenergic bronchodilators?
        a. Asthma
        b. Cystic fibrosis
        c. Chronic bronchitis
        d. Pulmonary fibrosis

11. The drugs known as adrenergic bronchodilators are all analogs of which naturally occurring neurotransmitter?
        a. Acetylcholine
        b. Norepinephrine
        c. Epinephrine
        d. Dopamine

12. Single-isomer $\beta_2$ agonists include which of the following?
        a. Salmeterol
        b. Levalbuterol
        c. Terbutaline
        d. microNefrin

13. In relation to bronchodilators, "rescue" agents refer to:
        a. Short-acting agents
        b. Long-acting agents
        c. Controllers
        d. Prodrugs

14. Which of the following is *not* a catecholamine?
        a. Isoetharine
        b. Isoproterenol
        c. Dopamine
        d. Terbutaline

15. Adrenergic bronchodilators have two isomers. Which of the following is the active isomer on airway $\beta_2$ receptors?
    a. The (R)-isomer, also called the levo isomer
    b. The (R)-isomer, also called the dextro isomer
    c. The (L)-isomer, also called the levo isomer
    d. The (L)-isomer, also called the dextro isomer

16. Which of the following statements concerning epinephrine is *not* true?
    a. It is a catecholamine.
    b. It stimulates both $\alpha$ and $\beta$ receptors.
    c. It is metabolized by cholinesterase.
    d. The natural form has only one isomer.

17. Which of the following statements concerning isoproterenol is *not* correct?
    a. It is a catecholamine.
    b. It stimulates both $\alpha$ and $\beta$ receptors.
    c. It is metabolized by COMT.
    d. It exists with two isomers.

18. Catecholamines are unsuitable for oral administration because of which of the following?
    a. Severe side effects
    b. The need for a megadose
    c. Their acidic pH
    d. Inactivation by the gut and liver

19. Exposure to which of the following does not readily inactivate catecholamines?
    a. Pressure
    b. Heat
    c. Light
    d. Air

20. Which of the following drugs is a saligenin?
    a. Terbutaline
    b. Isoetharine
    c. Alupent
    d. Albuterol

21. Which of the following drugs comes in an MDI formula that is breath activated?
    a. Tornalate
    b. Maxair
    c. Xopenex
    d. Foradil

22. Which of the following drugs is referred to as a prodrug?
    a. Advair
    b. Tornalate
    c. Xopenex
    d. Serevent

23. The only single-isomer short-acting bronchodilator available in the U.S. market is:
    a. Xopenex
    b. Severent
    c. Tornalate
    d. Maxair

24. A peak plasma concentration of Severent is seen 5 minutes after inhalation, with a second peak at 45 minutes. The second peak is the result of which of the following?
    a. Drug modification in the plasma
    b. Vascular absorption from the conduction airways
    c. Absorption of swallowed drug
    d. Metabolism by hydroxylation

25. To assess maximal response to albuterol, pulmonary function (peak flow or $FEV_1$) should be measured how many minutes after treatment?
    a. 5 minutes
    b. 15 minutes
    c. 45 minutes
    d. 120 minutes

26. Which of the long-acting bronchodilators also has a quick onset of action?
    a. Formoterol
    b. Salmeterol
    c. Metaproterenol
    d. Pirbuterol

27. Catecholamine bronchodilators are *not* available in which of the following forms?
    a. MDI
    b. Nebulizer solution
    c. Tablets
    d. Parenteral

28. Which of the following statements concerning desensitization with use of bronchodilators is *not* correct?
    a. It is caused by reduction in the number of $\beta$ receptors.
    b. The effect stabilizes within a few weeks with continued use.
    c. The desensitization is considered clinically important.
    d. Corticosteroids can reverse the desensitization.

29. Which of the following statements regarding the drop in $PaO_2$ after bronchodilator administration by inhalation is *not* true?
    a. It occurs because of ventilation–perfusion mismatch.
    b. The drop is physiologically significant.
    c. The drop is statistically significant.
    d. The drop in $SaO_2$ is minimal.

30. The general indication for adrenergic bronchodilators is to:
    a. Reduce the consistency of mucus
    b. Reduce inflammation
    c. Reduce blood flow to target organs
    d. Reverse or lessen the degree of airflow obstruction

31. Which of the following is *not* a symptom that occurs with administration of a catecholamine?
    a. Tachycardia
    b. Reduced blood pressure
    c. Bronchodilation
    d. Relaxation of skeletal smooth muscle vessels

32. Epinephrine is a potent catecholamine bronchodilator; in addition, it also has which of the following effects?
    a. $\alpha$ only
    b. $\beta_1$ only
    c. $\alpha$ and $\beta_1$
    d. $\beta_2$ only

33. A pediatric patient has stridor and has been diagnosed with croup. To help reduce the swelling in the upper airway, which drug would be most beneficial?
    a. Racemic epinephrine
    b. Terbutaline
    c. Isoetharine
    d. Levalbuterol

34. Albuterol has which of the following actions?
    I. Duration up to 6 hours
    II. $\beta_2$ preferential
    III. Peak effect within 30–60 minutes
    IV. Can be delivered by mouth
        a. I and II only
        b. II and III only
        c. I, II, and III only
        d. I, II, III, and IV

35. Which of the following is *not* a strength of Xopenex nebulized solution (in milligrams)?
    a. 1.25
    b. 0.63
    c. 0.31
    d. 0.05

36. Salmeterol is a _____-receptor agonist?
    a. $\alpha$ only
    b. $\alpha$ and $\beta_1$ only
    c. $\beta_2$ only
    d. $\alpha$, $\beta_1$, and $\beta_2$

37. This drug is used for prevention of acute exercise-induced bronchospasm in adults and children older than 12 years of age:
    a. Salmeterol
    b. Levalbuterol
    c. Albuterol
    d. Formoterol

38. National guidelines recommend the introduction of salmeterol to treat asthma at which level of care?
    a. Step 3
    b. Step 1
    c. Step 2
    d. Step 4

39. Asthmatics must be educated in the use of:
    a. Short-acting bronchodilators
    b. Long-acting bronchodilators
    c. Both long-acting and short-acting bronchodilators
    d. Long-acting bronchodilators and glucocorticoids

40. The Advair Diskus inhaler is a combination product of
    a. Salmeterol and fluticasone
    b. Salmeterol and albuterol
    c. Salmeterol and levalbuterol
    d. Salmeterol and epinephrine

41. Which of the following is *not* a reason why inhalation is the preferred route of administration of a $\beta$-adrenergic drug?
    a. Rapid onset
    b. Larger dose required as compared with the oral route
    c. Reduced side effects
    d. Painless and safe

42. A practical approach to optimal drug dosing in a patient brought to the emergency department with severe airway obstruction, and who does not respond to intermittent nebulizer treatments after 1 hour, would be

_____ _____ of β agonists.
   a. Increasing dosage
   b. Oral administration
   c. Subcutaneous injection
   d. Continuous nebulization

43. A respiratory therapist tells the physician that he is measuring the bronchodilating effect of a β agonist. The therapist would be:
   a. Determining the reaction of the airway by cold air introduction.
   b. Determining the reaction of the airway by the amount of wheezing produced by methacholine challenge
   c. Measuring airflow changes by measuring $FEV_1$
   d. Determining the reaction of the airway by introduction of histamine

44. Which of the following should be assessed to determine the benefit of long-acting β agonists in an asthmatic patient?
   I. Nocturnal symptoms
   II. Number of exacerbations
   III. Unscheduled clinic or hospital visits
   IV. Days of absence from work due to symptoms
       a. I and II only
       b. II and III only
       c. I, II, and IV only
       d. I, II, III, and IV

A 16-year-old patient suffers from moderate asthma. He is receiving a regimen of cromolyn sodium and corticosteroid.

1. What would be the best choice of sympathomimetic bronchodilator to accompany this therapy?

2. What is the one condition in which the sympathomimetic bronchodilator you chose in question 1 would be likely to cause your patient problems?

# 7 Anticholinergic (Parasympatholytic) Bronchodilators

## CHAPTER OBJECTIVES

*After answering the following questions, the reader should be able to:*

1. Differentiate between *parasympathomimetic* and *parasympatholytic*
2. Differentiate between *cholinergic* and *anticholinergic*
3. Differentiate between *muscarinic* and *antimuscarinic*
4. List all available anticholinergic agents used in respiratory therapy
5. Discuss the indication for anticholinergic agents
6. Explain the mode of action for anticholinergic agents
7. Describe the route of administration available for anticholinergic agents
8. Discuss adverse effects for anticholinergic agents
9. Discuss the clinical application for anticholinergic agents

## KEY TERMS AND DEFINITIONS

*Complete the following questions by writing the answer in the space provided.*

1. An agent that blocks parasympathetic nervous fibers is called _____.

2. An agent that produces the effect of acetylcholine is called _____.

3. An agent that blocks parasympathetic nervous fibers, which allow relaxation of smooth muscle in the airway, is

   called a(n) _____  _____.

4. _____ is the same as cholinergic, producing the effect of acetylcholine or an agent that

   mimics acetylcholine.

5. The word _____ has the same meaning as anticholinergic: blocking the effect of

   acetylcholine at the cholinergic site.

6. A _____ agent produces effects similar to those of the parasympathetic nervous system.

## CLINICAL INDICATIONS FOR USE

*Complete the following questions by writing the correct term in the blank provided.*

7. List two anticholinergic bronchodilators that are indicated as a bronchodilator for maintenance and treatment in chronic obstructive pulmonary disease (COPD), including chronic bronchitis and emphysema.

   a. _____

   b. _____

8. A combination of _____ and _____ is indicated for use in patients needing regular treatment for COPD, and who require additional bronchodilation for relief of airflow obstruction.

9. What two drugs make up Combivent?

   a. _____

   b. _____

10. The drug used in severe asthma, especially bronchoconstriction that does not respond well to β-agonist therapy,

   is _____.

## SPECIFIC ANTICHOLINERGIC (PARASYMPATHOLYTIC) AGENTS

*Complete the following questions by writing the correct term in the blank provided.*

11. List the brand names for the following. (*Hint:* Review Table 7-1 in the textbook.)

   a. Tiotropium bromide: _____

   b. Ipratropium bromide: _____

   c. Ipratropium bromide and albuterol: _____

12. Match the administration method to the correct drug.

   1. _____ Metered dose inhaler (MDI)

   2. _____ Hydrofluoroalkane (HFA) MDI

   3. _____ Nasal spray

   4. _____ Small volume nebulizer (SVN)

   5. _____ Dry powder inhaler (DPI)

   a. Atrovent
   b. Combivent
   c. DuoNeb
   d. Spiriva

13. Complete the following table for inhaled anticholinergic bronchodilator agents.

| | Adult Dosage | Time Course |
|---|---|---|
| Atrovent MDI | | |
| Atrovent HFA MDI | | |
| Combivent | | |
| DuoNeb | | |
| Spiriva | | |

14. Ipratropium bromide is a derivative of _____ _____ .

15. Atropine is a _____ _____

_____ and not fully ionized, and is therefore readily absorbed into the blood stream, is distributed throughout the body, crosses the blood–brain barrier, and causes changes in the CNS.

16. Ipratropium bromide (Atrovent) is a _____ _____

_____ and fully ionized. It is poorly absorbed, does not cross the blood–brain barrier, and does not cause CNS changes.

17. Considering the differences between tertiary and quaternary ammonium compounds, which type do you think has greater systemic side effects?

*Remember:* In asthma, ipratropium lasts about as long as a β agonist; but in COPD, ipratropium lasts 1 to 2 hours longer.

## PHARMACOLOGICAL EFFECTS OF ANTICHOLINERGIC (ANTIMUSCARINIC) AGENTS

18. Identify the following cholinergic effects and anticholinergic effects by marking an (X) in the appropriate box.

| | Cholinergic Effect | Anticholinergic Effect |
|---|---|---|
| Decreased heart rate | | |
| Drying of upper airway | | |
| Salivation | | |
| Mucociliary drying | | |
| Secretion of mucus | | |
| Bronchoconstriction | | |
| Inhibition of bronchial constriction | | |
| Increased heart rate | | |

19. Identify the pharmacological effects of tertiary and quaternary anticholinergic agents in the following table by placing an (X) in the appropriate box.

| | Tertiary (e.g., Atropine) | Quaternary (e.g., Ipratropium) |
|---|---|---|
| Bronchodilation | | |
| Blocks hypersecretion | | |
| No change in mucociliary clearance | | |
| Slowing of heart rate with small dosage, increased heart rate with large dosage | | |
| No heart rate effect | | |
| Blocks nasal hypersecretion | | |
| Decreased mucociliary clearance | | |

## MODE OF ACTION

Parasympathetic neurons from the vagus nerve enter the lung at the hila and travel along the airways. Parasympathetic postganglionic fibers terminate on or near the airway epithelium, submucosal glands, smooth muscle, and probably mast cells. Parasympathetic innervation and muscarinic receptors are concentrated in the larger airways, although present from the trachea to the respiratory bronchioles.

Normally a basal level of bronchomotor tone is caused by some parasympathetic activity. Administration of an anticholinergic abolishes this tone (allows bronchodilation), and administration of a parasympathomimetic intensifies the tone (causes bronchoconstriction). The degree of bronchodilation that will occur with anticholinergics depends on the degree of tone present, which is the result of parasympathetic stimulation. If parasympathetic stimulation is causing significant bronchoconstriction, then administration of an anticholinergic should result in significant bronchodilation.

*Complete the following question by writing the correct term in the blank provided.*

20. Methacholine, used in bronchial provocation testing to intensify the level of bronchial tone to the point of

bronchial constriction, would be a(n) _____ agent.

### Vagally Mediated Reflex Bronchospasm

Sensory C-fiber nerves respond to a variety of stimuli such as irritant aerosols, cold air, cigarette smoke, noxious fumes, and inflammatory mediators. When stimulated, they send an afferent nerve impulse to the CNS. This results in a reflex cholinergic efferent nerve impulse that results in bronchoconstriction, increased secretions, and cough. The anticholinergic agents block this parasympathetic reflex response.

21. The most common side effects seen with anticholinergic aerosol ipratropium are

_____  _____ and _____.

22. True or False: The nebulized dose of ipratropium is more than 10 times greater than the MDI dose, which causes greater systemic side effects.

*The following questions concern delivery of a quaternary ammonium antimuscarinic bronchodilator such as ipratropium bromide. Identify each statement as either true or false.*

23. True or False: Patients must use a holding chamber with MDI administration.

24. True or False: With nebulizer delivery, the patient must be instructed to keep the mouthpiece in the mouth, and a reservoir tube should be attached to the expiratory side of the T mouthpiece facing away from the patient.

25. True or False: Facemask delivery is recommended in order to deliver the maximal dose of the drug.

## CLINICAL APPLICATION

26. Complete the following table by comparing the general clinical effects of anticholinergic and β-adrenergic bronchodilators. (*Hint:* Review Table 7-5 in the textbook.)

| | Anticholinergic | β Agonist |
|---|---|---|
| Onset | | |
| Time to peak effect | | |
| Duration | | |
| Fall in $Pao_2$ | | |
| Site of action | | |

### Use in Chronic Obstructive Pulmonary Disease

Anticholinergic bronchodilators seem to have their greatest effect on the central airways. They are more potent bronchodilators than β-adrenergic bronchodilators in the bronchitis–emphysema combination. This is their primary clinical application.

27. The U.S. Food and Drug Administration (FDA) has given approval for ipratropium specifically for use in the

treatment of _____.

Inhaled antimuscarinic agents have been found to be more potent bronchodilators than β-adrenergic agents in patients with COPD. Antimuscarinics have a slightly slower onset of action and peak effect, but their duration of action is as long or longer than that of most β agonists. Tiotropium bromide offers some exciting possibilities. It has a prolonged duration of action (up to 24 hours) and maintains lung function at a higher level than ipratropium. It may have a significant effect on quality of life and reduce breathlessness in patients with COPD.

### Use in Asthma

Anticholinergic bronchodilators aren't really better than β-adrenergic bronchodilators in the treatment of asthma. But they might be useful if the patient has side effects with another class of bronchodilator or if patients need to be treated with β blockers (patients with hypertension).

28. Beside improving lung function in COPD and controlling symptoms, tiotropium may also be useful for controlling

_____ _____ symptoms and deterioration of flow rates at nighttime.

29. Anticholinergics may be useful in patients with acute severe episodes of asthma not responding to

_____.

## COMBINATION THERAPY: β-ADRENERGIC PLUS ANTICHOLINERGIC AGENTS

The combination of β-adrenergic agents and anticholinergic agents could provide a one–two punch for patients with COPD or asthma.

30. Anticholinergics act primarily on the _____ airways; β agonists act primarily on the

   _____ airways.

31. True or False: Because albuterol peaks sooner and terminates sooner, and ipratropium peaks slowly and lasts longer, they complement each other.

32. In a large, controlled study COPD patients given a combination of albuterol and ipratropium showed a greater

   increase in _____ compared with patients given either agent alone.

Although parasympathetic nerve fibers are found from the trachea to the respiratory bronchioles, they are concentrated in the larger, central airways. This is where the anticholinergic agents exert most of their effect. β-Agonist bronchodilators exert their effect in both the large and small airways. When giving two separate drugs, which should be given first? It probably doesn't matter. If the patient has a preference, let him decide. Many times these drugs are given as a combination drug mixture, so there is no choice.

33. Combination drug mixtures (albuterol and ipratropium) include _____ and

   _____.

## RESPIRATORY CARE ASSESSMENT OF ANTICHOLINERGIC BRONCHODILATOR THERAPY

*Circle True or False for the following statements:*

34. True or False: Administration of an anticholinergic bronchodilator therapy requires assessing pulse during treatment and after treatment.

35. True or False: Pulmonary function studies of lung volumes, capacities, and flows are required for long-term management.

36. True or False: It is important to instruct the patient in the use of small volume nebulizers at home but not in the use of MDIs or DPIs, because the latter are simple to understand and use.

37. True or False: Assessing the number of exacerbations, unscheduled clinic visits, and hospitalizations would be helpful to determine the effectiveness of a long-acting antimuscarinic bronchodilator.

## NATIONAL BOARD OF RESPIRATORY CARE–TYPE QUESTIONS

Hasn't time flown since we began this chapter? I know you're shocked to learn that NBRC questions are next.

1. An agent that blocks parasympathetic nervous fibers, which allow relaxation of airway smooth muscle, is called:
   a. Parasympatholytic
   b. An anticholinergic bronchodilator
   c. Muscarinic
   d. Cholinergic

2. A physician has written an order to give a patient Combivent; the order provides no other information. How many puffs and how often should the patient receive this treatment?
   a. 2 puffs, qid
   b. 2 puffs, once per day
   c. 2 puffs, bid
   d. 2 puffs, q4h

3. A patient calls the pulmonary rehabilitation department and tells the therapist that she has been taking Spiriva twice per day for the past 2 days. The respiratory therapist should tell the patient to:
   a. Continue on this routine
   b. Increase the treatment to three times per day
   c. Take the medication once per day
   d. Increase the treatment to four times per day

4. The total adult dose of Atrovent HFA MDI after one treatment would be:
   a. 17 µg
   b. 34 µg
   c. 39 µg
   d. 100 µg

5. A drug with cholinergic effects would *not* result in which of the following?
   a. Decreased heart rate
   b. Salivation
   c. Secretion of mucus
   d. Increased heart rate

6. A parasympathomimetic agent that intensifies the level of bronchial tone to the point of bronchial constriction and is used in bronchial provocation testing is:
   a. Atropine
   b. Ipratropium
   c. Methacholine
   d. Tiotropium

7. Beside improving lung function in COPD and controlling symptoms, tiotropium may also be useful for controlling symptoms and deterioration of flow rates with:
   a. Nocturnal asthma
   b. Nonexacerbation of acute bronchitis
   c. Chronic bronchitis
   d. Exercise-induced asthma

8. Which of the following could be assessed to determine the effectiveness of tiotropium bromide?
   I. Keep account of the number of exacerbations
   II. Keep account of the number of unscheduled clinic visits
   III. Keep account of the amount of sputum expectorated during exacerbations
   IV. Keep account of the number of hospitalizations
   a. I and II only
   b. II and III only
   c. I, II, and IV only
   d. I, II, III, and IV

9. Anticholinergic agents competitively block the action of which of the following substances?
   a. Catechol
   b. Sympathomimetics
   c. β-Adrenergic agents
   d. Acetylcholine

10. Which of the following is *not* true of tertiary ammonium compounds?
    a. An example is ipratropium bromide.
    b. An example is atropine.
    c. They are associated with more CNS side effects than are quaternary ammonium compounds.
    d. They are associated with more cardiac side effects than are quaternary ammonium compounds.

11. Which of the following describes quaternary ammonium compounds?
    a. They cross the blood–brain barrier.
    b. The are easily absorbed.
    c. They do not cause CNS changes.
    d. They are distributed throughout the body.

12. Combivent is a combination of which of the following drugs?
    a. Metaproterenol and atropine
    b. Albuterol and atropine
    c. Metaproterenol and ipratropium
    d. Albuterol and ipratropium

13. Which is most effective in the treatment of COPD?
    a. Anticholinergic agents
    b. β-Adrenergic agents
    c. Alternate-day therapy
    d. Both a and b

14. In comparing anticholinergic and β-adrenergic agents, anticholinergic agents are associated with which of the following:
    a. Faster onset
    b. Quicker time to peak effect
    c. No development of tolerance
    d. Shorter duration of action

15. If ipratropium is delivered as an aerosol nebulizer treatment with a mask, what precautions should be taken?
    a. Pinch the nose of the patient.
    b. Stand outside the room.
    c. Caution the patient not to swallow.
    d. Protect the patient's eyes.

Jane has a 100 pack-year smoking history. She suffers from a combination of emphysema and chronic bronchitis. Lately, she's been more short of breath than usual, and her dyspnea is accompanied by some expiratory wheezing. What do you think she'll respond to better—sympathomimetic bronchodilators or anticholinergic bronchodilators?

# 8 | Xanthines

## CHAPTER OBJECTIVES

*After answering the following questions, the reader should be able to:*

1. Define *xanthine*
2. List all available xanthines used in respiratory therapy
3. Differentiate between the clinical indications and uses of xanthines
4. Discuss the proposed theories of activity for xanthines
5. Discuss adverse effects and toxicity of xanthines
6. Be able to clinically assess xanthine therapy

Nobody is sure how xanthines work, which makes it nice for you (there's less to learn)! Xanthines are generally thought of as second- or third-string drugs in treating asthma and chronic obstructive pulmonary disease (COPD).

## CLINICAL INDICATIONS FOR USE OF XANTHINES

*Complete the following questions by writing the answer in the space provided, or by providing a brief answer.*

1. For the treatment of acute exacerbations of asthma, _____ are *not* generally recommended.

2. Why is theophylline recommended only as an alternative to inhaled bronchodilators in the treatment of COPD?

3. Why is caffeine citrate used with premature infants?

4. Why might caffeine citrate be used in preference to theophylline with premature infants?

## SPECIFIC XANTHINE AGENTS

*Complete the following questions by writing the correct term in the space provided.*

5. List three types of methylxanthines.

   a. _____

   b. _____

   c. _____

6. List three available formulations of theophylline.

a. _____

b. _____

c. _____

## GENERAL PHARMACOLOGICAL PROPERTIES

The following lists the physiological effects of xanthines. These are easy to remember if you associate them with how you feel after drinking a large coffee, or Mountain Dew:

- CNS stimulation
- Cardiac muscle stimulation
- Cerebral vasoconstriction
- Diuresis
- Bronchial and vascular smooth muscle relaxation
- Peripheral and coronary vasodilation
  Theophylline and caffeine, although exerting the same effects, do so to varying extents.

7. Identify the intensity of effects for caffeine and theophylline, using the following symbols: +++, most intense; ++, less intense; +, least intense.

| Effect | Caffeine | Theophylline |
|---|---|---|
| CNS stimulation | | |
| Smooth muscle relaxation | | |
| Skeletal muscle stimulation | | |
| Cardiac stimulation | | |
| Diuresis | | |

8. In the treatment of asthma and COPD, rank the following classes of bronchodilators from most to least effective (1 is most effective):

| Treatment of Asthma | Treatment of COPD |
|---|---|
| a. Anticholinergic agents: _____ | a. Anticholinergic agents: _____ |
| b. β Agonists: _____ | b. β Agonists: _____ |
| c. Xanthines: _____ | c. Xanthines: _____ |

## PROPOSED THEORIES OF ACTIVITY

The exact method of action of the xanthines is unknown. Originally it was thought that the xanthines inhibited phosphodiesterase, allowing increased levels of intracellular cyclic AMP and bronchodilation. However, this pathway has been doubted because of the low drug levels used in humans. A second possibility is that theophylline blocks the action of adenosine, which when present can lead to bronchoconstriction. This proposal is also a weak argument. A third explanation is that xanthines cause the release of endogenous catecholamines, but conflicting results have been reported. Other theories include inhibition of calcium uptake and an antagonizing effect on prostaglandins. This brings us back to the beginning: the exact method of action of the methylxanthines is unknown.

## TITRATING THEOPHYLLINE DOSES

People metabolize theophylline at different rates, so it's difficult to determine a therapeutic dose. In addition, different forms of the drug aren't always equivalent, making it even more difficult.

The optimal serum theophylline level for maximal bronchodilation in adults is believed to be between 10 and 20 µg/ml.

9. Given the following levels of serum theophylline, indicate the effect each level has on the body.

| Micrograms (mg)/milliliter (ml) | Effect |
|---|---|
| a.  <5 | |
| b.  10 to 20 | |
| c.  >20 | |
| d.  >30 | |
| e.  40 to 45 | |

Since the 10- to 20-µg/ml range for theophylline was proposed 25 years ago, it has been narrowed somewhat for the treatment of asthma and COPD.

10. A range of _____ µg/ml is now recommended for the treatment of asthma, and a range of

_____ µg/ml is recommended for the treatment of COPD.

11. What happens if the serum level of theophylline is too low?

12. What would you recommend as a course of action if a patient's serum level of theophylline were too low?

## DOSAGE SCHEDULES

Because of the variable rate at which people metabolize theophylline, dosage schedules are used to titrate it.

13. After a patient has been administered theophylline (assume you have properly calculated the dose), your patient complains of nausea. What would you suggest?

Dosage of theophylline should be guided by clinical reactions *and* serum drug levels.

14. After administering an immediate-release form of theophylline, serum blood levels should be obtained

_____ to _____ hours later.

15. After administering a sustained-release form of theophylline, serum blood levels should be measured

_____ to _____ hours after the morning dose.

## THEOPHYLLINE TOXICITY AND SIDE EFFECTS

Theophylline has a narrow therapeutic margin and distressing side effects can be seen even when serum levels are within the therapeutic range. The most common adverse reactions with theophylline use are listed in Box 8-1 in the textbook. Adverse reactions can be unpredictable, with little warning given before serious side effects occur.

16. Match the adverse reactions seen with theophylline with the organ system.

1. _____ Diuresis

2. _____ Tachypnea

3. _____ Nausea

4. _____ Anxiety

5. _____ Palpitations

6. _____ Vomiting

7. _____ Headache

a. CNS
b. Gastrointestinal
c. Respiratory
d. Cardiovascular
e. Renal

17. What precautions might you take when administering theophylline to patients with bronchiectasis or cystic fibrosis?

## FACTORS AFFECTING THEOPHYLLINE ACTIVITY

18. Circle the correct response: Theophylline is metabolized by the (liver/kidney) and excreted by the (liver/kidney).

Theophylline also interacts with other drugs. These drug interactions, along with any condition that affects the liver or kidneys, can have effects on the serum level of theophylline. Box 8-2 in the textbook lists some of the drugs and conditions that influence (increase or decrease) theophylline serum levels. This, in turn, affects dosing. When factors affecting theophylline levels are present, it is very important to monitor serum levels. Theophylline and β agonists have an additive effect. Theophylline may antagonize the sedative effect of valium and reverse the paralyzing effect of nondepolarizing neuromuscular blocking agents.

*Identify each of the following statements as either true or false.*

19. True or False: Theophylline can be used for maintenance therapy in COPD if ipratropium bromide and β agonists can't control the disease.

20. True or False: As far as asthma is concerned, the American Thoracic Society suggests that theophylline be used only to provide relief *after* β agonists, corticosteroids, and prophylactic agents have been implemented to target the underlying inflammation.

21. True or False: Long-acting $\beta_2$ agonists such as salmeterol may be used to preserve lung function in COPD before using theophylline.

22. True or False: According to the Global Initiative for Chronic Obstructive Lung Disease (GOLD) guidelines, intravenous aminophylline should not be used to manage acute exacerbation of COPD.

23. True or False: A nonbronchodilating effect of theophylline is its ability to directly strengthen the diaphragm.

24. True or False: Theophylline decreases cardiac output and increases pulmonary vascular resistance, thus potentially imposing a greater work load on the heart.

25. True or False: When treating apnea of prematurity it is better to use theophylline than caffeine because theophylline is a more potent stimulator of the respiratory system.

26. True or False: Serum concentrations of caffeine of 5–20 mg/L have been effective in treating apnea of prematurity.

## NATIONAL BOARD OF RESPIRATORY CARE–TYPE QUESTIONS

As if this news isn't wonderful enough, the NBRC questions are next!

1. Theophylline is chemically referred to as one of which of the following?
   a. β Blockers
   b. Anticholinergics
   c. Methylxanthines
   d. Aminophylline agonists

2. Xanthines exhibit all of the following physiological effects *except:*
   a. Bronchial smooth muscle relaxation
   b. Cerebral vasodilation
   c. Coronary vasodilation
   d. Diuresis

3. Compared with the β agonists, theophylline has what degree of bronchodilating effect?
   a. Weak
   b. Comparable
   c. Strong
   d. Very strong

4. Which of the following make it difficult to titrate theophylline doses?
   I. Theophylline has a short half-life.
   II. Individuals metabolize theophylline at different rates.
   III. Different forms of theophylline are not always equivalent.
   IV. The therapeutic range varies widely between patients.
      a. I, II, and III only
      b. II and III only
      c. II and IV only
      d. I, III, and IV only

5. In the management of asthma, the therapeutic range for serum theophylline is which of the following?
   a. 2 to 12 µg/ml
   b. 5 to 15 µg/ml
   c. 20 to 30 µg/ml
   d. >30 µg/ml

6. Cardiovascular side effects associated with theophylline use include all but which of the following?
   a. Hypotension
   b. Ventricular dysrhythmias
   c. Supraventricular tachycardia
   d. Atrial dysrhythmias

7. Nonbronchodilating effects of theophylline include all of the following *except:*
   a. Increased diaphragmatic strength
   b. Increased phrenic nerve activity
   c. Increased pulmonary vascular resistance
   d. Increased cardiac output

8. Theophylline may be used to treat all but which of the following?
   a. Pneumonia
   b. Apnea of prematurity
   c. COPD
   d. Asthma

9. In which of the following situations are methylxanthines generally *not* recommended for use?
   a. Acute exacerbations of asthma
   b. Maintenance therapy for mild persistent asthma
   c. Acute exacerbations of COPD
   d. Stable COPD

10. The methylxanthines are considered first-line agents in the treatment of:
    a. Congestive heart failure
    b. Asthma
    c. COPD
    d. Apnea of prematurity

11. In which of the following formulations is theophylline *not* available?
    a. Oral
    b. IV
    c. Aerosol
    d. Rectal suppository

12. Why is caffeine considered the drug of choice, compared with theophylline, for treatment of apnea of prematurity?
    I. It penetrates more readily into the cerebrospinal fluid.
    II. It is a more potent stimulator of the CNS.
    III. It has a higher therapeutic index.
    IV. It has fewer side effects.
       a. I and II only
       b. II and III only
       c. I, III, and IV only
       d. I, II, III, and IV

13. The exact mechanism of action of the methylxanthines is:
    a. Inhibition of phosphodiesterase
    b. Antagonism of adenosine
    c. Release of catecholamines
    d. Unknown

14. The recommended serum level for theophylline when treating COPD is:
    a. 0-5 µg/ml
    b. 5-15 µg/ml
    c. 10-12 µg/ml
    d. 10-20 µg/ml

15. A serum blood theophylline level of 27 µg/ml has been determined for an adult patient in the emergency department. Which of the following effects may be seen with this serum level?
    a. No effects
    b. Cardiac arrhythmias
    c. Nausea and vomiting
    d. Seizures

16. Before using theophylline, which of the following drugs would be of greater benefit as a maintenance agent for COPD?
    I. Salmeterol
    II. Albuterol
    III. Ipratropium bromide
    IV. Caffeine
       a. I only
       b. II and IV only
       c. I, II, and III only
       d. I, III, and IV only

17. A serum concentration of _____ mg/L of caffeine has been found effective in treating apnea of prematurity.
    a. 0.5-1
    b. 3
    c. 1-4
    d. 5-20

18. A patient with bronchiectasis has been taking theophylline for several days. She notices that her secretions are more difficult to expectorate and are much thicker. On the basis of these findings you would:
    a. Instruct her to drink more fluids
    b. Reduce the concentration of theophylline
    c. Determine the serum level of theophylline
    d. Switch theophylline to caffeine

19. With which of the following does theophylline *not* have an antagonistic effect?
    a. Valium
    b. Pancuronium
    c. Albuterol
    d. None of the above

Joe has been recently diagnosed with COPD. He is 57, has worked in the coal mines since he was 17, and suffers from severe dyspnea. Joe's physician prescribed oxygen for home use at 2 L/min, β agonists, and corticosteroids. Joe has not responded as his physician had hoped. (There has been no change in his forced expiratory volume in 1 second [$FEV_1$]). Joe's physician has decided to initiate sustained-release theophylline, and asks you to calculate the appropriate dose for Joe. He weighs 75 kg and is 6 feet tall.

1. What dose should Joe begin with?

The following day Joe calls his physician and states that he feels no improvement. The doctor suggests to Joe that he will increase his dose but he will need to check his theophylline level first.

2. When is the best time to do this?

His serum level comes back as 5 μg/ml. Joe still feels no change or improvement since starting the medication.

3. What should be recommended?

# 9 Mucus-Controlling Drug Therapy

## CHAPTER OBJECTIVES

*After answering the following questions, the reader should be able to:*

1. Interpret the physiology and mechanisms of mucus secretion and clearance
2. Name the types of mucoactive medications and their presumed modes of action
3. Describe the medications approved for the therapy of mucus clearance disorders and their approved indications
4. Identify the contraindications to the use of mucoactive medications
5. Explain the interaction between airway clearance devices or physical therapy and mucoactive medications

## KEY TERMS AND DEFINITIONS

*Match the following definitions with their terms.*

1. _____ A macromolecular description of pseudo-plastic material having both viscosity and elasticity

2. _____ A medication that increases ciliary clearance of respiratory mucus secretions

3. _____ The deformation and flow (strain) of matter

4. _____ A medication meant to increase the volume or hydration of airway secretions

5. _____ This is the principal constituent of mucus

6. _____ A rheologic property characteristic of liquids and represented by the loss modulus *G*

7. _____ A medication that degrades polymers in secretions

8. _____ Secretion, from surface goblet cells and submucosal glands, composed of water, proteins, and glycosylated mucins

9. _____ A term connoting any medication or drug that has an effect on mucus secretion

10. _____ Expectorated secretions that contain respiratory tract, oropharyngeal, and nasopharyngeal secretions as well as bacteria and products of inflammation including polymeric DNA and actin

a. Elasticity
b. Expectorant
c. Gel
d. Mucin
e. Mucoactive agent
f. Mucokinetic agent
g. Mucolytic agent
h. Mucoregulatory agent
i. Mucospissic
j. Mucus
k. Rheology
l. Sputum
m. Viscosity

11. _____ A drug that reduces the volume of airway mucus secretion and appears to be especially effective in hypersecretory states such as bronchorrhea, diffuse panbronchiolitis (DPB), cystic fibrosis (CF), and some forms of asthma

12. _____ A rheologic property characteristic of solids; it is represented by the storage modulus $G'$

13. _____ A medication that increases the viscosity of secretions and may be effective in the therapy of bronchorrhea

## DRUG CONTROL OF MUCUS: A PERSPECTIVE

The mucociliary escalator is one of the major defense mechanisms of the lung, with many lung diseases being associated with abnormal mucociliary function. It is suggested that drugs used in respiratory care be called mucoactive agents instead of mucolytics, which implies a breaking down of mucus. The major goal of mucoactive therapy is to reduce the accumulation of airway secretions, and this should be considered after taking steps to decrease mucus production. These steps include decreasing airway irritation and infection.

14. The term *mucolytic*, indicating breakdown of mucus, is better replaced with _____ agent.

15. For the three mucoactive agents listed, provide the following information:

| Drug | Brand Name | Use | Adult Dose |
|------|-----------|-----|-----------|
| *N*-Acetylcysteine 10% | | | |
| Dornase alfa | | | |
| Aqueous aerosols: | | | |
| water, saline | | | |

## PHYSIOLOGY OF THE MUCOCILIARY SYSTEM

Mucus lines several areas of the body, including the airways, and seems to provide protective services including lubrication, waterproofing, and antibacterial activity. Airway mucus has two layers: the outer, or gel, layer that is "firmer" and moves toward the larynx and the inner, or sol, layer in which the cilia are bathed. The inner watery layer is also referred to as the periciliary layer. The secretory structures that contribute to these layers include the ciliated epithelial cells and surface goblet cells, in a ratio of 5:1, and Clara cells and submucosal glands. The submucosal glands have both serous and mucous cells. The submucosal glands are thought to provide the majority of mucus secretion. Their mucus is transported to the airway surface by ciliated ducts.

Mucus is made up of secretions from the mucous membranes. Sputum, on the other hand, includes mucus, secretions from the upper airway, and other material such as bacteria, products of inflammation, and particulate matter.

Mucociliary transport occurs as a result of the beating cilia. There are approximately 200 cilia per cell, moving at a rate of 660 to 1080 beats/min (11 to 18 beats/sec). They are approximately 7 μm in length in large airways and 5 μm in smaller bronchioles. Mucus moves at an estimated rate of 1.5 mm/min in the lung periphery and 20 mm/min in the trachea. A surfactant layer lies at the tip of the cilia, separating the sol and gel layers. This allows the cilia to move the gel layer without becoming entangled in it. Mucus transport rates slow in the presence of chronic obstructive pulmonary disease (COPD), atropine, narcotics, endotracheal suctioning, cigarette smoke, atmospheric pollutants, and with both hyperoxia and hypoxia.

16. True or False: Drinking milk will increase respiratory tract congestion due to increases in mucus production.

## NATURE OF MUCUS SECRETION

A healthy individual produces about 100 ml of mucus per day, of which approximately 10 ml reaches the glottis. The volume can be dramatically increased in disease states. Mucus is a complex macromolecule referred to as a *glycoprotein*. The flexible strands of mucus cross-link, incorporate water, and form a gelatinous matrix. Once formed, little topical water is incorporated. This may help explain why some aerosolized solutions have been ineffective in "thinning" secretions. Ion transport across the epithelial cells lining the airway helps regulate the amount and composition of the periciliary fluid level. Dysfunction of the ion channels, as in cystic fibrosis, can lead to abnormal amounts and consistency of mucus. In general, airway disorders promote increased mucus amounts and viscosity, slowed ciliary motion, bronchial obstruction, increased airflow resistance, and atelectasis.

17. Complete the following table concerning the effects of various drug groups on mucociliary clearance.

| Drug Group | Ciliary Beat | Mucus Production |
|---|---|---|
| β Adrenergic agents | | |
| Cholinergic agents | | |
| Methylxanthines | | |
| Corticosteroids | | |

18. True or False: Approximately 10 ml of secretions reaches the glottis of the 100 ml produced from the lungs each day.

## MUCUS IN DISEASE STATES

The normal clearance of airway mucus can be altered by changes in the volume, hydration, or composition of the secretion. Mucus is produced and secreted by surface goblet cells and submucosal gland cells. Water content is a function of transepithelial chloride secretion, active sodium absorption, and water transport. Knowledge of these features of respiratory mucus may lead to a better understanding of diseases characterized by an abnormal production of mucus such as chronic bronchitis and asthma, where there is mucus hypersecretion, and CF, where there is decreased mucus secretion.

19. _____ _____ is considered the most important predisposing factor to airway irritation and mucus hypersecretion, but other factors can include viral infections, pollutants, and genetic predisposition in patients with chronic bronchitis.

20. True or False: β Agonists induce the secretion of viscous mucus, so it is possible that in acute severe asthma, the aggressive use of β agonists may contribute to fatal airway obstruction.

21. Cystic fibrosis (CF) is associated with chronic airway infection, often with _____ and other gram-negative organisms.

22. The secretions in CF have very little _____ are almost entirely composed of

_____ _____ derived from neutrophil degradation.

## PHYSICAL PROPERTIES OF MUCUS

Let's review—again—several terms used to describe the physical properties of mucus.

*Adhesion* is the frictional force between mucus and the airway surface. Increased adhesion severely limits the ability to clear mucus when coughing. *Viscosity* is a measure of the resistance of a fluid to flow. An increase in mucus viscosity slows the mucociliary escalator. *Elasticity* is a measure of the ability of a deformed material to return to its original shape. *Spinnability* describes the ability of mucus to be drawn out into long threads.

Normal mucus has a relatively low viscosity and high elasticity and spinnability. Purulent sputum has increased viscosity and decreased spinnability, which impedes mucus transport.

23. Why is it so difficult for a person with purulent sputum to cough it up?

## MUCOACTIVE AGENTS

Other than bronchodilators, the only approved mucoactive agents are both mucolytics. *N*-Acetylcysteine disrupts disulfide bonds, whereas dornase alfa enzymatically breaks down DNA in airway secretions. These mucolytics decrease the viscosity and elasticity of secretions. Decreased viscosity promotes mucus clearance, whereas decreased elasticity may actually have a negative effect on mucus clearance.

## MUCOLYTICS

Mucolytic agents decrease the elasticity and viscosity of mucus by breaking down the gel structure. Because elasticity is crucial for mucociliary transport, mucolytics have the potential for a negative effect on normal physiological mucus clearance. Reduction of mucus gel to a more liquid state may facilitate aspiration of secretions with the use of suction catheters.

24. Discuss two therapeutic options, beside using mucoactive agents, for controlling mucus hypersecretion.

### *N*-Acetyl-L-Cysteine (NAC)

As a respiratory agent, NAC is mucolytic in action. Despite demonstrating *in vitro* mucolytic activity, there are no data that clearly show that aerosolized NAC is an effective therapy. NAC works by disrupting disulfide bonds and is more effective in alkaline pH environments (7.0 to 9.0). The most serious hazard of using NAC is bronchospasm due to its acidity. Predosing or simultaneous delivery of a rapid-acting bronchodilator with NAC can lessen the chance of this complication. Other complications include nausea, runny nose, and oral cavity inflammation. Because it has been shown to be ineffective in pulmonary disorders, it should not be used to treat patients with pulmonary disorders. The "rotten egg" odor is due to the release of hydrogen sulfide. NAC is incompatible in solution with some antibiotics, and they should not be mixed together for aerosolization. NAC also can be used as an oral antidote for acetaminophen (Tylenol) overdose to help prevent hepatic injury.

25. NAC works by disrupting _____ _____ and is more effective in alkaline pH environments (7.0 to 9.0).

26. When administering NAC by aerosol bronchospasm may occur. The incidence of bronchospasm can be reduced by

pretreatment with a _____-_____ bronchodilator.

27. True or False: A light purple color indicates NAC has expired and should be discarded.

28. True or False: NAC can be used to treat acetaminophen (Tylenol) overdose and is administered orally.

### Dornase Alfa

Dornase alfa (Pulmozyme) is a clone of a natural human enzyme. It is manufactured by using genetically engineered Chinese hamster ovary cells. Initially called rhDNase, Pulmozyme is approved for use in patients with cystic fibrosis (CF) who have tenacious respiratory secretions. Pulmozyme is an orphan drug. (Remember, from Chapter 1, that an *orphan drug* is one used for rare diseases, with *rare* defined as fewer than 200,000 cases in the United States; a drug may also be designated an orphan if it is used for a disease that affects more than 200,000 persons but there is no reasonable expectation of recovering the costs of drug development.)

Chronic respiratory infections in patients with CF cause migration of large numbers of neutrophils to the airway. After fighting infection, they are destroyed and release their DNA. The DNA adds bulk to the secretions and increases the viscosity of the sputum. Aerosolized Pulmozyme breaks down the DNA, reducing viscosity and adhesiveness, thus helping to mobilize secretions. Common side effects with the use of Pulmozyme include voice alteration, inflammation of the upper airway, a rash, chest pain, and eye inflammation.

The only contraindication to dornase alfa is hypersensitivity to the drug. The beneficial effect of dornase alfa may not be in any great improvement in lung function but instead may be in the decreased number and severity of pulmonary infections. This would result in decreased use of antibiotics and fewer hospitalizations.

29. Why should dornase alfa not be prescribed for subjects with bronchiectasis and COPD?

30. List two indications for dornase alfa:

    a. _____

    b. _____

31. What nebulizers and compressors have been approved for delivery of dornase alfa?

32. Why is it important to nebulize dornase alfa with the recommended nebulizer systems?

33. How would you evaluate the effectiveness of dornase alfa with a CF patient?

### *F*-Actin–Depolymerizing Drugs: Gelsolin and Thymosin $\beta_4$

Chronic inflammation is characterized by inflammatory cell necrosis and release of undegraded DNA, filamentous actin (F-actin), and intracellular enzymes from neutrophils. These are present in patients with CF. Gelsolin has been shown to reduce the viscosity of sputum in CF sputum.

## EXPECTORANTS

- SSKI, a supersaturated solution of potassium iodide, is thought to stimulate secretion of airway fluids.
- Sodium bicarbonate (2%), a weak base, has been directly instilled into the trachea and aerosolized to increase local pH and weaken bonds in mucus.
- Guaifenesin may stimulate the cholinergic pathway and increase mucus secretion from the submucosal glands.
- Oligosaccharides disrupt hydrogen bonds in mucin. Dextran also may have an osmotic effect that increases mucus hydration. Aerosolized heparin has shown promise in the treatment of asthma.

These and other expectorants have shown little clinical effectiveness.

## MUKOKINETIC AGENTS

### β Agonists

β Agonists (discussed earlier) increase ciliary beat frequency and increase expiratory airflow by dilating airways. In some patients with "floppy airways," as in bronchiectasis, this airway muscle relaxation can also decrease expiratory airflow by producing dynamic airway collapse. β Agonists are also mucus secretagogues and therefore may increase mucus plugging if they increase dynamic collapse and decrease expiratory airflow.

34. What disease would benefit from increased expiratory airflow with the use of β agonists?

## SURFACE-ACTIVE PHOSPHOLIPIDS

Surfactant is produced in alveoli and in the conducting airways. A thin layer exists between the gel and sol layers of mucus, at the tip of the cilia. This layer helps prevent airway dehydration, promotes mucus spreading, and improves mucociliary transport. In the absence of surfactant, mucus sticks to the epithelium, rendering cough less effective. There is severe loss of surfactant in the inflamed airway of patients with chronic bronchitis or CF. Surfactant aerosol improves pulmonary function and sputum transportability in patients with chronic bronchitis or with CF, and this effect is dose dependent.

35. What two diseases have shown improvement with administration of aerosolized surfactant?

## MUCOREGULATORY MEDICATIONS

Another approach to reducing the burden of airway secretions is to decrease hypersecretion by goblet cells and submucosal glands. Anticholinergic medications are also extensively used as mucoregulatory medications. Atropine is routinely given perioperatively to prevent laryngospasm and to decrease mucus secretion associated with endotracheal intubation. Atropine and its derivatives are mucoregulatory medications in that they do not "dry" secretions but will decrease hypersecretion that is mediated through $M_3$ cholinergic mechanisms. The quaternary ammonium derivatives of atropine, including ipratropium bromide and tiotropium, do not significantly cross the blood–airway barrier and, as such, their use is not associated with typical systemic effects of anticholinergic medications such as flushing or tachycardia.

36. The long-term use of a mucoregulatory medication such as ipratropium is associated with a reduction in the

volume of mucus secretion in patients with _____ _____.

## ANTIPROTEASES

Neutrophils release proteases (elastase) that damage epithelial cells. They also cause significant production of secretions from the submucosal glands. Intravenous administration or inhalation of $\alpha_1$-antitrypsin suppresses the activity of neutrophil elastase and restores the bacteria-killing capacity of neutrophils.

37. In what disease would antiproteases be helpful in restoring the bacteria-killing capacity of neutrophils?

## HYPEROSMOLAR SALINE

For many years, sputum induction produced by hyperosmolar saline inhalation has been used to obtain specimens for the diagnosis of pneumonia. Long-term use of inhaled hyperosmolar saline improves pulmonary function in patients with CF. Although this therapy is readily available and inexpensive, hypertonic saline aerosol is not as effective as dornase alfa in the therapy of CF lung disease. Furthermore, hypertonic saline has an unpleasant taste and induces coughing; these features may limit its acceptance and hence its efficacy as a long-term therapy.

38. A CF patient has been prescribed hyperosmolar therapy using a 6% hypertonic saline solution administered bid. What delivery device should be used for this therapy?

## USING MUCOACTIVE THERAPY WITH PHYSIOTHERAPY AND AIRWAY CLEARANCE DEVICES

A number of physical factors affect secretion clearance. Cephalad airflow bias is responsible for the movement of mucus in airways during normal ventilation. The narrowing of airways on exhalation increases the velocity and shearing forces in the airway, creating a cephalad airflow bias with tidal breathing. This bias is amplified during coughing, when increased transmural pressure causes the airways to fold and constrict, increasing airflow velocity even further.
*Identify each of the following statements as either true or false.*

39. True or False: Conventional chest physiotherapy (CPT) incorporating postural drainage results in significantly greater expectoration than no treatment in patients with cystic fibrosis.

40. True or False: The insufflation–exsufflation device inflates the lungs with positive pressure followed by a negative pressure to simulate a cough.

41. True or False: The active cycle of breathing techniques utilizes relaxed diaphragmatic breathing and the insufflation–exsufflation device.

42. True or False: Autogenic drainage incorporates staged breathing, starting with small tidal breaths from expiratory reserve volume (ERV), repeated until secretions "collect" in the central airways. It is recommended for patients >8 years of age.

43. True or False: Exercise, if tolerated, should be substituted for other bronchial hygiene regimens.

44. True or False: Positive airway pressure (PAP) techniques can be effective alternatives to chest physical therapy in expanding the lungs and mobilizing secretions. Pursed-lip breathing is an example.

45. True or False: High-frequency chest wall compression (HFCWC) increases tracheal mucus clearance rates and correlates with improved ventilation, thus increasing mucus clearance.

*Complete the following questions by writing the correct term in the space provided.*

46. What device combines PEP with high-frequency oscillations at the airway opening?

47. With what airway clearance device does the patient breathe through a mouthpiece that delivers high-flow minibursts at rates exceeding 200 cycles/min?

48. Which airway clearance device provides pressure pulses that fill a vest and vibrate the chest wall at variable frequencies applied during the entire respiratory cycle?

## NATIONAL BOARD OF RESPIRATORY CARE–TYPE QUESTIONS

Now, practice with the following NBRC-type questions.

1. A mucokinetic medication is one that:
   a. Increases ciliary clearance of respiratory mucus secretions
   b. Increases the volume or hydration of airway secretions
   c. Degrades polymers in secretions
   d. Increases ciliary activity

2. Pulmozyme is used primarily for:
   a. Chronic bronchitis
   b. Sputum induction
   c. Cystic fibrosis
   d. Bronchitis

3. How would you evaluate the effectiveness of dornase alfa in the CF patient?
    I. Reduction in IV antibiotic use
    II. Reduced need for hospitalizations
    III. Stability of lung function
    IV. Reduced number and severity of infectious exacerbations
        a. I, II only
        b. III, IV only
        c. I, III, IV only
        d. I, II, III, IV

4. Which of the following is *not* one of the layers of mucus?
    a. Glycoprotein
    b. Periciliary
    c. Surfactant
    d. Gel

5. Which of the following cells or glands is most likely responsible for the majority of mucus secretion?
    a. Ciliated epithelial cells
    b. Goblet cells
    c. Clara cells
    d. Submucosal glands

6. Which of the following statements concerning submucosal glands is *not* correct?
    a. They are innervated by the parasympathetic nervous system.
    b. They are innervated by the sympathetic nervous system.
    c. They contain only serous secretory cells.
    d. Their secretions pass through ciliated ducts to the airway lumen.

7. Cilia beat at approximately what rate?
    a. 2 to 4 cycles/s
    b. 5 to 9 cycles/s
    c. 11 to 18 cycles/s
    d. 20 to 24 cycles/s

8. Which of the following forces severely reduces the ability to clear secretions by coughing?
    a. Viscosity
    b. Adhesion
    c. Elasticity
    d. Spinnability

9. All of the following drugs increase ciliary beat *except:*
    a. β Adrenergics
    b. Cholinergics
    c. Methylxanthines
    d. Corticosteroids

10. Which of the following is considered the most important predisposing factor to airway irritation and mucus hypersecretion with chronic bronchitis?
    a. Viral infections
    b. Tobacco smoke
    c. Pollutants
    d. Genetic predisposition

11. Cystic fibrosis (CF) is associated with chronic airway infection, often with:
    a. *Pseudomonas aeruginosa*
    b. *Staphylococcus aureus*
    c. *Streptococcus aureus*
    d. *Haemophilus influenzae*

12. Which of the following are therapeutic options for controlling mucus hypersecretion other than using mucoactive agents?
   I. Remove causative factors, such as pollution, where possible.
   II. Treat infections.
   III. Optimize tracheobronchial clearance, including the use of bronchodilators.
   IV. Incorporate bronchial hygiene measures such as cough and postural drainage.
      a. I and II only
      b. II and III only
      c. I, III, and IV only
      d. I, II, III, and IV

13. Which of the following is considered to be a mucoactive agent?
   I. Dornase alfa
   II. Acetylcysteine
   III. Budesonide
   IV. Sodium bicarbonate
      a. I and II only
      b. II and III only
      c. I, II, and IV only
      d. I, II, III, and IV

14. When administering NAC by aerosol it is important to include pretreatment with which of the following to reduce the incidence of bronchospasm?
   a. Rapid-onset bronchodilator
   b. Corticosteroid
   c. Cholinergic medication
   d. Expectorant

15. NAC, a mucoactive agent, reduces mucin by disrupting
   a. Beating cilia
   b. Neutrophilic action
   c. Disulfide bonds
   d. Protein synthesis

16. Opened vials of NAC should be stored in a refrigerator and discarded:
   a. When the NAC has turned a light purple color
   b. After 96 hours
   c. After 4 days whether vials have been opened or not
   d. When the NAC has turned pink

17. Which of the following is *not* suggested equipment for nebulization of dornase alfa?
   a. Hudson Updraft II
   b. Acorn II
   c. Pari LC Jet Plus
   d. Hamilton Fat Boy II

18. Common side effects with the use of Pulmozyme do *not* include:
   a. Voice alteration
   b. Inflammation of the upper airway
   c. Thrush
   d. Eye inflammation

19. For which disease would antiproteases be helpful in restoring the bacteria-killing capacity of neutrophils?
   a. Chronic bronchitis
   b. Emphysema
   c. ARDS
   d. CF

These aren't NBRC questions, but they're good practice.
*Match the descriptions to the appropriate airway clearance method.*

1. _____ Mr. Cilia is a 69-year-old COPD patient. He uses this positive airway pressure (PAP) technique as an effective alternative to chest physical therapy in expanding the lungs and mobilizing secretions.

2. _____ Randolph is a 32-year-old CF patient and uses this device when he is traveling. This device combines positive expiratory pressure (PEP) with high-frequency oscillations at the airway opening.

3. _____ Robin is a 29-year-old who has CF. She is a sales person for a pharmaceutical company and travels extensively and is very motivated. The airway clearance technique she uses incorporates staged breathing starting with small tidal breaths from ERV, repeated until secretions "collect" in the central airways. It is recommended for patients >8 years of age.

4. _____ Ronald is an 18-year-old with CF and he is attending his first year of college away from home. Because he is independent and must perform his own therapy the airway clearance device he uses provides pressure pulses that fill a vest and vibrate the chest wall at variable frequencies applied during the entire respiratory cycle. He uses it for 20–30 minutes per treatment and takes his nebulized medication at the same time.

5. _____ Alfred is a 22-year-old and has CF. He does not tolerate or like any other device except for this one, which provides breaths through a mouthpiece and delivers high-flow minibursts at rates exceeding 200 cycles/min.

6. _____ Mary is a 44-year-old with cerebral palsy. She has poor coughing and limited expiratory airflow. When in the hospital she uses this device, which can generate high-frequency oscillations at the airway opening or on the chest wall.

7. _____ Lauren is 18 years old and has cerebral palsy and severe scoliosis. This device inflates her lungs with positive pressure followed by a negative pressure to simulate a cough.

8. _____ Jasmin has just taken a job as a traveling respiratory therapist. Jasmin has CF and feels it would be best to use a technique that allows her not to take equipment with her. Her CF clinic taught her this airway clearance technique. It is a combination of breathing control (relaxed diaphragmatic breathing), thoracic expansion control (deep breaths), and a forced expiration technique from progressively increasing lung volumes.

a. Chest wall oscillation: The Vest
b. Intrapulmonary percussive ventilation (Percussionator)
c. FLUTTER mucus clearance device
d. Autogenic drainage
e. Active cycle of breathing technique
f. An insufflation–exsufflation device
g. Pursed-lip breathing

Johnny is a 5-year-old recently diagnosed with cystic fibrosis. Dr. Pulmo has just met with Johnny and his parents. They have come to your office for you to instruct them in the respiratory care Johnny will be receiving and to answer any questions concerning his care. Dr. Pulmo has ordered albuterol, dornase alfa, and The Vest airway clearance system for Johnny. He is to return for a follow-up visit in 2 weeks.

1. The parents want to know what equipment they will need to deliver the dornase alfa and albuterol to Johnny and how often he should get it.

2. The parents know a CF child who is 13 years old and does autogenic drainage and percussion and postural drainage, which do not require equipment. Can Johnny be taught this now and use this instead of The Vest?

3. Are there any side effects associated with Pulmozyme? Albuterol?

4. The nurse gave the parents a chart with lung drainage positions. Because Johnny will use The Vest, does he need to be placed in these drainage positions while he is undergoing treatments?

5. How long should Johnny use The Vest in each treatment?

6. What if he doesn't tolerate or like The Vest? Can he switch to something else?

# 10 Surfactant Agents

## CHAPTER OBJECTIVES

*After answering the following questions, the reader should be able to:*

1. Define *surfactant*
2. List all available exogenous surfactant agents used in respiratory therapy
3. Describe the mode of action for exogenous surfactant agents
4. Discuss the route of administration for exogenous surfactant agents
5. Recognize hazards and complications of exogenous surfactant therapy
6. Assess the use of surfactant therapy

## KEY TERMS AND DEFINITIONS

*Complete the following questions by writing the answer in the space provided.*

1. A surface-active agent designed to lower surface tension is called a(n) _____.

2. The force caused by the attraction between like molecules, which occurs at liquid–gas interfaces, and which holds

   the liquid surface intact, is called _____ _____. The unit of
   measurement is dynes per centimeter (dyn/cm).

Because liquid molecules are more attracted to each other than they are to gas molecules, they sort of "draw in" on themselves, and a spherical shape is the result.

3. Laplace's Law describes and quantifies the relationship between

   a. _____

   b. _____

   c. _____

LaPlace's Law: pressure = (4 × surface tension)/radius, for a bubble. In the alveoli LaPlace's Law is as follows: pressure = (2 × surface tension)/radius.

4. Why is Laplace's Law different in the alveoli?

5. Therefore, as Laplace's Law applies to the lung, the _____ the surface tension the greater the

   compressing force inside the alveolus, which can lead to _____ of the alveolus.

6. Fill-in the following table of exogenous surfactant preparations currently approved in the United States.

| Drug | Brand Name | Amount in Vial | Initial Dose |
| --- | --- | --- | --- |
| Beractant | | | |
| Calfactant | | | |
| Poractant alfa | | | |

## EXOGENOUS SURFACTANTS

*Exogenous surfactant* refers to drugs that are preparations formed outside the patient's own body. The key to the use of exogenous surfactants is the recycling activity of surfactant production. More than 90% of surfactant is reabsorbed, processed, and secreted back onto the alveolar surface.

Natural surfactant is obtained from animals or humans and contains the necessary components for regulating surface tension. Natural surfactant can be expensive to prepare and may contain microbes (viruses) or antigens that may stimulate an immunological response. Natural surfactants are usually modified by addition or removal of components. Examples of natural surfactant include Survanta from minced cow (bovine) lung, Curosurf from pig (porcine) lung extract, and Infasurf from fluid extracted from calf (bovine) lung.

7. Exogenous surfactant is clinically indicated for the treatment and prevention of _____ in the newborn infant.

8. _____ treatment helps prevent RDS in very-low-birth-weight infants, and in higher birth weight infants who have evidence of immature lungs and who are at risk for developing RDS.

9. Circle the correct answer: In RDS, surface tension is abnormally (high, low).

### Composition of Pulmonary Surfactant

*Complete the following question by writing the answer in the space provided.*

10. What is the primary function of surfactant in the lung?

Pulmonary surfactant is made up of lipids (85% to 90%) and proteins (10%). (It's manufactured by type II alveolar cells, and its main function is to regulate surface tension of the liquid lining of the alveolus.)

11. Dipalmitoylphosphatidylcholine (DPPC), or _____, is primarily responsible for reduction of alveolar surface tension.

About 20% of the protein present is surfactant specific protein (SP). Four proteins have been identified: SP-A, SP-B, SP-C, and SP-D. SP-A regulates both secretion and exocytosis of surfactant from type II cells, as well as reuptake of surfactant into the type II cells. SP-B and SP-C improve the absorption and spreading of phospholipids throughout the alveoli. SP-D has no defined role in surfactant at this time.

The major stimulus for surfactant secretion appears to be lung inflation. The estimated alveolar half-life of surfactant is 15 to 30 hours. Clearance of surfactant is controlled by several mechanisms. Most surfactant is reabsorbed back into the type II cells for reuse through the process of endocytosis. Other clearance mechanisms include macrophage clearance, removal by mucociliary transport, and degradation.

12. Surfactant lipids are synthesized and stored in type II alveolar cells in vesicles termed _____

_____.

This is why only one or two doses of exogenous surfactant is usually required. It is taken into the surfactant pool and recycled as just described.

   Surfactant has been found to contribute to increased bacterial killing, improved macrophage function, decreased inflammatory response, and improved ciliary function.

   As a bonus, surfactant enhances ciliary beat frequency and helps maintain airway patency.

13. Addition of surfactant to an RDS lung will lower _____ _____ and

   increase lung _____.

14. What change has occurred to the pressure–volume curve in Figure 10-2 of your textbook after administration of surfactant to the RDS lung?

### Types of Exogenous Surfactant Preparations

*Complete the following questions by writing the answer in the space provided.*

15. _____ surfactants are obtained from animals or humans by alveolar wash or from amniotic fluid.

16. Survanta and Infasurf come from _____ lungs and Curosurf comes from

   _____ lungs.

What's good about natural surfactant: it's composed of the right materials to do the job. What's bad: it's expensive and time consuming to prepare, and contamination is a real concern. So what about synthetic surfactants? At present no synthetic surfactants are available.

### SPECIFIC EXOGENOUS SURFACTANT PREPARATIONS

*Complete the following questions by writing the answer in the space provided.*

17. What are two indications for the use of beractant (Survanta)?

   a. _____

   b. _____

18. How much Survanta should be given for prophylactic treatment of a newborn infant weighing 1000 g?

*Identify each of the following statements as either true or false.*

19. True or False: If a suspension of Survanta has settled, shake the vial for 30 seconds before administration.

20. True or False: Survanta must be refrigerated, but warmed for 20 minutes before administration.

21. True or False: A calculated dose of Survanta is administered through a 5-French catheter placed within the endotracheal tube.

22. True or False: After tracheal administration of the first dose of Survanta, the infant is placed back in the ventilator for 3-5 minutes before administering the next dose.

In summary, beractant (Survanta) is a modified natural surfactant. DPPC, palmitic acid, and tripalmitin are added to the bovine extract. The ingredients are suspended in normal saline in an 8-ml vial. Guidelines for the use of Survanta include both prophylactic and rescue treatment of infants with RDS. The recommended dose of Survanta is 4 ml/kg birth weight (100 mg of phospholipids). Beractant is light brown to off-white in color. Vials may be swirled gently to mix the contents, but they should not be shaken. Solutions should be refrigerated but warmed to room temperature for 20 minutes before delivery. Quarter-doses should be delivered through a 5-French catheter placed in the endotracheal tube (ETT). Ventilation for at least 30 seconds should be given between quarter-doses.

23. What are the indications for the use for calfactant (Infasurf)?

   a. _____

   b. _____

24. What is the recommended dose of Infasurf for an 800-g premature newborn infant?

25. True or False: Repeat doses of Infasurf, up to a total of three doses, can be given 12 hours apart.

26. True or False: Repeat doses of Infasurf as early as 6 hours after the previous dose can be given if the infant is still intubated and requires 30% or greater oxygen for an arterial oxygen pressure (PaO$_2$) of 80 mmHg or less.

27. What is the difference in patient positioning between side-port administration and catheter administration of Infasurf?
   Side-port administration:

   Catheter administration:

In summary, calfactant (Infasurf) is a modified natural surfactant that does not contain SP-A. Guidelines include instructions for both prophylactic and rescue treatment of infant RDS. The off-white suspension is ready for use and may be swirled for mixing but not shaken. The recommended dose is 3 ml/kg birth weight. Repeat doses of Infasurf as early as 6 hours after the previous dose can be given if the infant is still intubated and requires 30% or greater oxygen for an arterial oxygen pressure (PaO$_2$) of 80 mmHg or less. Administration can be by direct side-port ETT delivery or with the use of a catheter. Half-doses should be used for side-port administration and quarter-doses for catheter administration. Right and left side lying positions are used for half-dose administration, and four positions are used for catheter administration: prone, supine, right lateral, and left lateral.

28. List two indications for the use of poractant alfa (Curosurf)

    a. _____

    b. _____

29. What is the recommended initial dose of Curosurf for a newborn premature infant with a birth weight of 800 g?

30. True or False: After an initial dose of Curosurf subsequent doses of 1.25 ml/kg can be given twice at 12-hour intervals.

31. True or False: A vial of Curosurf should be shaken for 30 seconds to uniformly disperse the suspension.

32. True or False: A dose of Curosurf is administered through a 5-French catheter not to be extended beyond the end of the endotracheal tube.

33. True or False: If significant airway obstruction occurs with Curosurf dosing the airway can be suctioned.

34. True or False: After administration of each dose of Curosurf the catheter is removed and the infant is manually ventilated with 100% oxygen for 1 minute.

35. Describe how an infant is positioned during administration of Curosurf.

In summary, poractant alfa (Curosurf) is a natural surfactant. Guidelines for use include treatment or rescue of infants with RDS and unlabeled uses include severe meconium aspiration syndrome (MAS) and respiratory failure caused by group B streptococcal (GBS) infection. Dosage is 2.5 ml/kg birth weight with subsequent doses of 1.25 ml/kg at 12-hour intervals (maximum of 5 ml/kg, initial plus repeat doses). The suspension should be delivered at room temperature, using a catheter, and in two half-doses. The infant should be positioned on the right side for one half-dose and on the left side for the other. The suspension can be turned upside down to mix the suspension but should not be shaken.

## HAZARDS AND COMPLICATIONS OF SURFACTANT THERAPY

Because you are delivering relatively large volumes of suspension to tiny airways, gas exchange may be blocked, causing desaturation and/or bradycardia.

As a result of delivery of exogenous surfactant, pulmonary compliance should improve. This may result in the following:

- Overventilation: This may require reducing pressure with pressure-limited, time-cycled ventilation, reduction in volume with pressure-regulated, constant-volume, or volume-guaranteed ventilation, alteration in ventilator rate, or adjustment in baseline pressures.
- Hyperoxygenation with high $Pao_2$ levels, which can contribute to retrolental fibroplasia (retinopathy of prematurity).

36. List three observations that would indicate that a newborn infant has responded well to administration of exoge-
    nous surfactant:

    a. _____

    b. _____

    c. _____

## NATIONAL BOARD OF RESPIRATORY CARE–TYPE QUESTIONS

It's time for some NBRC-type questions.

1. Surfactant accomplishes which of the following?
   a. Decreases lung compliance
   b. Lowers surface tension
   c. Forces pulmonary blood flow to perfuse nonventilated alveoli
   d. Improves mucociliary escalator

2. Which of the following happens as the surface tension of the liquid lining of the alveolus increases?
   a. More pulmonary blood flow perfuses the alveoli.
   b. It becomes more difficult for the alveolus to inflate.
   c. Airway resistance decreases.
   d. More type I cells are produced.

3. Surfactant is produced by which type of alveolar cell?
   a. Type I
   b. Type II
   c. Type III
   d. Macrophage

4. Which of the following describes surfactant preparations from outside the patient's own body?
   a. Endogenous
   b. Mysogenous
   c. Exogenous
   d. Detergent-type

5. Surfactant is composed of which of the following?
   a. A variety of amino acids
   b. 10% lipids and 90% proteins
   c. 50% lipids and 50% proteins
   d. 90% lipids and 10% proteins

6. How is exogenous surfactant administered?
   a. Aerosol route
   b. Direct instillation into the trachea
   c. IV
   d. Parenteral route

7. Which of the following is LaPlace's Law as it relates to the alveoli?
   a. $4 \times$ surface tension/radius
   b. $4 \times$ radius/surface tension
   c. $2 \times$ radius/surface tension
   d. $2 \times$ surface tension/radius

8. What would be the initial dose of Infasurf administered for prophylactic treatment of a newborn infant weighting 1 kg?
   a. 3.5 ml in four divided doses
   b. 3.0 ml in two divided doses
   c. 2.5 ml in four divided doses
   d. 5.0 ml in two divided doses

9. What is the primary function of surfactant in the lung?
   a. To regulate surface tension force of the liquid lining of the alveoli
   b. To regulate pulmonary artery blood flow to the alveoli
   c. To increase alveolar ventilation by reducing airway resistance
   d. To regulate the mucociliary escalator to improve secretion clearance

10. Which of the following is primarily responsible for reduction of alveolar surface tension?
    a. Sphingomyelin
    b. Surfactant protein D
    c. Lecithin
    d. Surfactant protein A

11. The major stimulus for surfactant secretion is believed to be:
    a. Baroreceptors
    b. Chemoreceptors
    c. Pulmonary artery blood flow
    d. Lung inflation

12. Which of the following is *not* true concerning Survanta?
    a. The suspension should not be shaken to mix it.
    b. After refrigeration it should be warmed for 20 minutes.
    c. The calculated dose is administered through a side-port on the endotracheal tube adaptor.
    d. The initial dose is 4 ml/kg divided into four equal aliquots.

13. Prophylactic Infasurf treatment is indicated for:
    a. Term infants with MAS
    b. Infants <29 weeks of gestational age at risk for developing RDS
    c. Infants with GBS pneumonia
    d. Infants >72 hours of age at risk for developing RDS

14. A respiratory therapist is about to administer Infasurf by intratracheal catheter. Appropriate positioning of the infant includes:
    a. Prone position for all doses
    b. Right and left side dependent following each dose
    c. Supine position for all doses
    d. Different positioning following each dose: prone, supine, right and left dependent

15. Which of the following procedures should occur immediately after administration of Survanta through a 5-French catheter?
    a. The patient should be turned to the opposite side and the second dose administered.
    b. On removal of the catheter the infant should be manually ventilated for 30 seconds.
    c. On removal of the catheter the infant should be manually ventilated for 2–5 minutes.
    d. On removal of the catheter the infant should be placed back on mechanical ventilation in the prone position.

16. Two hours after administration of exogenous surfactant an infant receiving mechanical ventilation shows an increase in exhaled tidal volume, from 5 to 9 ml/kg of body weight, with no change in pressure delivery. These findings would indicate:
    a. Reduced airway resistance
    b. Increased lung compliance
    c. Increased work of breathing
    d. The need to administer another dose of surfactant

17. An intubated infant just received 1.0 ml of Survanta through a 5-French catheter. The infant is being hand venti-lated with 90% oxygen. Suddenly the infant's heart rate drops from 140 to 75 beats/min, $SpO_2$ (oxygen saturation as determined by pulse oximetry) decreases from 89 to 70%, and work of breathing and retractions increase. The respiratory therapist should make which of the following recommendations:
    a. Extubate and manually ventilate the infant.
    b. Turn the infant so the opposite lung is dependent.
    c. Suction the endotracheal tube.
    d. Reconnect the infant to the ventilator.

18. The respiratory therapist reports to the physician that an infant has had a good response to administration of Curosurf, as indicated by:
    I. Increase in $Pao_2$
    II. Increase in $Spo_2$
    III. Increase in lung compliance
        a. I only
        b. II and III only
        c. I and III only
        d. I, II, and III

19. Natural surfactant is obtained from:
    I. Lungs of cows
    II. Lungs of pigs
    III. Lungs of pigeons
        a. I only
        b. I and II only
        c. II and III only
        d. I, II, and III

20. Survanta rescue treatment of infants with evidence of RDS should occur:
    a. Within 8 hours of birth
    b. Immediately after birth
    c. Within 2 hours of birth
    d. Within 1 hour of birth

21. How much Survanta should be administered for prophylactic treatment of a newborn weighing 700 g?
    a. 2.8 ml
    b. 2.1 ml
    c. 4.0 ml
    d. 4.2 ml

A male newborn infant with a gestational age of 26 weeks and a birth weight of 900 g is in the neonatal intensive care unit (NICU). The 4-hour-old infant is intubated and has been receiving mechanical ventilation since birth. The decision has been made to administer Survanta. This baby fits the protocol's inclusion criteria, and you have been asked to talk to the parents about this decision.

1. How would you explain to the parents what RDS is and why exogenous surfactant is needed?

2. The parents would like to know how you would determine whether their child is getting better after administration of the surfactant?

After talking with you, the parents consent to the treatment. You return to the NICU and prepare to administer Infasurf.

3. After removing the vial of Infasurf from the refrigerator, how long will it take for the vial to warm to room temperature?

4. You notice that settling has occurred within the vial. How should it be mixed?

5. How much of the 8-ml vial will the infant require for the first dose?

6. How would you administer Infasurf through a side-port on the endotracheal tube adaptor?

7. You return to the parents and explain the procedure to them. They ask, "What will happen if he doesn't get better? Can he get more surfactant?" What is your answer?

# 11 Corticosteroids in Respiratory Care

## CHAPTER OBJECTIVES

*After answering the following questions, the reader should be able to:*

1. Discuss the indications for inhaled corticosteroid use
2. List all available inhaled corticosteroids used in respiratory therapy
3. Differentiate between specific corticosteroid formulations
4. Describe the route of administration available for corticosteroids
5. Describe the mode of action for corticosteroids
6. Discuss the effect corticosteroids have on the white blood cell count
7. Discuss the effect corticosteroids have on β receptors
8. Differentiate between systemic and local side effects of corticosteroids
9. Discuss the use of corticosteroids in the treatment of asthma and chronic obstructive disease
10. Be able to clinically assess corticosteroid use in patient care

## KEY TERMS AND DEFINITIONS

*Complete the following questions by writing the answer in the space provided.*

1. The hyperglycemia resulting from steroids increasing plasma glucose levels through the breakdown of proteins is

   called _____ _____.

2. Substances, such as corticosteroids, produced within the body are called _____.

3. A gamma globulin produced by cells in the respiratory tract is _____.

4. This hormone-type substance, an inflammatory mediator and part of the arachidonic acid cascade, is called

   _____.

5. Also known as glucocorticoids, _____ produce an antiinflammatory response in the body.

6. Chemicals secreted by the adrenal cortex, and referred to as steroids, are called _____

   _____ _____.

7. Substances produced outside the body, for administration inside the body, are called _____.

8. Inflammatory process chemicals, produced and released by the body in response to stimuli, are called

   _____ _____.

*Complete the following questions by writing the answer in the space provided.*

9. List two formulations in which inhaled corticosteroids are available.

   a. _____

   b. _____

10. At what level of care in asthma, as defined by the National Asthma Education and Prevention Program (NAEPP) Expert Panel Report 2 *Guidelines for the Diagnosis and Management of Asthma—Update on Selected Topics*, are corticosteroids clinically indicated?

11. In severe asthma both inhaled corticosteroids and _____ corticosteroids can be used together.

12. List two clinical indications for intranasal aerosolized corticosteroids:

   a. _____

   b. _____

13. Match the following aerosolized corticosteroids for oral inhalation with their brand name.

| Drug | Brand Name |
|------|------------|
| a. ____ Triamcinolone acetonide | 1. AeroBid, AeroBid-M |
| b. ____ Budesonide | 2. QVAR |
| c. ____ Beclomethasone dipropionate HFA | 3. Pulmicort Turbuhaler |
| d. ____ Fluticasone propionate/salmeterol | 4. Azmacort |
| e. ____ Flunisolide | 5. Advair Diskus |
| f. ____ Budesonide/formoterol fumarate | 6. Symbicort |

14. Match the following aerosolized corticosteroids for intranasal delivery with their brand name.

| Drug | Brand Name |
|------|------------|
| a. ____ Triamcinolone acetonide | 1. Nasonex |
| b. ____ Beclomethasone | 2. Beconase AQ |
| c. ____ Flunisolide | 3. Rhinocort Aqua |
| d. ____ Fluticasone | 4. Flonase |
| e. ____ Budesonide | 5. Nasarel |
| f. ____ Mometasone furoate monohydrate | 6. Nasocort AQ |

## PHYSIOLOGY OF CORTICOSTEROIDS

### Identification and Source

Corticosteroids are a group of chemicals secreted by the adrenal cortex. They're called adrenal cortical hormones. The adrenal gland has two parts:
   1. Inner zone: Produces epinephrine
   2. Outer zone: Produces corticosteroids

The corticosteroids used in pulmonary disease are all derivatives of cortisol, also known as hydrocortisone.

It is important to understand how the body produces and controls its own corticosteroids. The release of endogenous steroids is controlled by the hypothalamic–pituitary–adrenal (HPA) axis. Stimulation of the HPA axis results in release of steroids. In general, steroids regulate metabolism to increase levels of glucose for body energy. One of the most significant side effects of using exogenous steroids is HPA suppression. Normally, when endogenous steroids are released, there is a feedback mechanism that limits their production. When exogenous steroids are administered, they block or suppress the release of the endogenous steroids. This effect can be seen 1 day after the administration of systemic steroids. Methods delivering aerosolized steroids do not deliver enough drug to replace the missing endogenous steroid. Therefore, any time a patient is being switched from systemic to aerosolized steroids, the systemic administration must be weaned slowly until the body can resume its normal endogenous production.

15. List two side effects of glucocorticoid drugs:

a. _____

b. _____

Endogenous glucocorticosteroid production follows a daily 24-hour cycle referred to as a *diurnal* or *circadian rhythm*. Usually, steroid levels are highest in the morning and taper throughout the day. One treatment option to help decrease the side effects of exogenous steroid therapy is to give the steroids on alternate days and early in the morning. This timing allows increased levels to occur at the time when the body would normally have increased levels. The alternate-day therapy allows the body's own system to resume production on the day the exogenous steroid is not given.

16. One of the primary reasons for using aerosolized glucocorticoids is to minimize _____ suppression.

17. To withdraw an adrenally suppressed patient from oral corticosteroid treatment, the oral agent is tapered off slowly

while _____ corticosteroids are started.

## NATURE OF THE INFLAMMATORY RESPONSE

Inflammation is the response of vascularized tissue to injury. The triple response usually involves redness, flare, and wheal. These include increased vascular permeability, leukocyte infiltration, phagocytosis, and mediator release.

Lung inflammation can be caused by several factors including trauma, inhalation of noxious substances, infections, and allergic responses. Asthma and chronic bronchitis are the two most common inflammatory lung diseases seen. Asthma is a disease with chronic airway inflammation. Along with the inflammatory response already noted, airway inflammation results in smooth muscle contraction (bronchospasm), increased mucus production, shedding of airway cells, and goblet cell hyperplasia. Clinical signs and symptoms include wheezing, breathlessness, chest tightness, and coughing. Glucocorticosteroids are a mainstay in the prevention and treatment of the inflammatory response; they inhibit the activity of inflammatory cells and the mediators of inflammation.

18. Name two of the most common inflammatory lung diseases:

a. _____

b. _____

19. Give a description of each category of the triple response to inflammation:

a. _____

b. _____

c. _____

## INFLAMMATION IN THE AIRWAY

Corticosteroids reduce inflammation: it is that simple. Asthma is a disease characterized by chronic inflammation of the airway and hyperresponsiveness to various stimuli.

Mast cells and eosinophils are the major players in causing the inflammatory response. The mediators that are released during an asthma attack cause bronchoconstriction, edema, and increased secretions.

20. There is evidence that the early asthmatic response is caused by _____-dependent activation of airway mast cells.

Treatment with antiinflammatory agents such as glucocorticoids is important to reduce the basal level of airway inflammation in asthma, thereby reducing airway hyperresponsiveness and the predisposition to acute episodes of obstruction. Bonus effects of glucocorticoids include suppression of plasma leakage and mucus secretion in inflamed airways, and restoration of responsiveness to β-adrenergic stimulation.

21. List three bonus effects of glucocorticoids in the treatment of asthma:

    a. _____

    b. _____

    c. _____

## AEROSOLIZED CORTICOSTEROIDS

22. Many of the corticosteroid aerosol agents have transitioned from chlorofluorocarbon (CFC)-propelled metered

    dose inhaler (MDI) formulations to _____.

Review Tables 11-1 and 11-2 in the textbook for aerosol corticosteroid preparations available for oral inhalation and intranasal delivery. Drug strength and doses for adults and children are listed in these tables.

23. Beclomethasone dipropionate (QVAR), which was known as Vanceril and Beclovent, has been reformulated with a

    hydrofluoroalkane (HFA) propellant; it has a lung deposition measured at _____% to

    _____% of the emitted dose.

24. Triamcinolone acetonide (Azmacort) and flunisolide (AeroBid, AeroSpan) are marketed with a built-in

    _____ device.

25. Flunisolide shows a peak plasma level after inhalation between 2 and 60 minutes, indicating good

    _____ from the lungs.

26. Flovent HFA is the _____ form and Flovent Diskus is the _____ form of fluticasone propionate.

27. What is the benefit of using budesonide in the form of Pulmicort Respules as compared with the Pulmicort Turbuhaler?

28. What two drugs are contained within the DPI Advair?

29. What two drugs make up Symbicort?

All the steroids available as orally inhaled agents are also available in an intranasal formulation. See Table 11-2 in the textbook for a listing of these intranasal formulations.

## PHARMACOLOGY OF CORTICOSTEROIDS

Glucocorticoids inhibit many of the cells involved in airway inflammation including macrophages, T lymphocytes, eosinophils, and mast cells. They also cause microvasculature contraction to decrease leakage of fluid into the inflammatory sites. Glucocorticoids are lipophilic (they move easily through lipid membranes) and enter cells to bind to steroid receptors. There are three general pathways by which steroids suppress the inflammatory response:

1. Increased (upregulated) transcription of antiinflammatory genes for antiinflammatory proteins (e.g., lipocortin)
2. Suppression of factors that cause gene transcription involved with inflammation (e.g., nuclear factor-$\kappa$B)
3. Increased (upregulated) expression of inhibitors that suppress gene expression for proinflammatory proteins (e.g., cytokines)

Another benefit of steroids is their ability to restore responsiveness to $\beta$-adrenergic stimulation, something that is often lost during acute asthmatic episodes. This is accomplished by increasing the number and availability of $\beta$ receptors and their affinity for $\beta$ agonists. Research also has shown that steroids prolong the action of endogenous catecholamines.

Glucocorticoids inhibit many cells that are involved in airway inflammation, such as macrophages, T lymphocytes, eosinophils, and mast cells, and reverse the shedding of epithelial cells and goblet cell hyperplasia seen in asthma.

30. The _____ _____ _____ count increases in patients taking glucocorticoids systemically.

Sometimes, in the midst of an asthma attack, a patient is no longer responsive to $\beta$ agonists. Glucocorticoids restore that responsiveness; this effect can happen 1 to 4 hours after IV administration of glucocorticoids. So if you see a bolus of steroid being administered to an asthmatic patient who is doing poorly, it's being done to restore responsiveness to $\beta$ agonists.

31. Give one reason for administering a bolus of glucocorticoids in status asthmaticus.

## HAZARDS AND SIDE EFFECTS OF STEROIDS

The following is a list of a few of the side effects associated with systemic administration of corticosteroids. Others can be found in Box 11-3 in the text.

- Immunosuppression resulting in increased susceptibility to infection
- Fluid retention resulting from sodium-sparing effects of glucocorticoids
- Increased white blood cell count with an increase in neutrophils and decrease in lymphocytes and eosinophils
- Hypertension resulting from fluid retention
- Dermatological changes leading to cushingoid appearance (moon face)
- Hyperglycemia from reduced glucose uptake

32. Immunosuppression, caused by systemic use of steroids, can lead to susceptibility to infection by

_____, _____, or _____ agents.

### Systemic and Local Side Effects With Aerosol Administration

Although corticosteroids have far fewer side effects when they're given by aerosol, side effects do occur. The higher the dose (of inhaled corticosteroids), the greater the possibility that the patient will experience side effects. Also, if a patient is switched from systemic to inhaled administration, the patient may experience adrenal insufficiency, extrapulmonary allergy, or acute asthma; so wean the patient gradually from oral to inhaled administration.

33. Circle the correct answer: Potential systemic hazards and side effects with inhaled aerosol corticosteroids include (adrenal insufficiency/dysphonia).

34. What are the two most common side effects caused by topical application of inhaled steroids?

a. _____

b. _____

35. List three ways to minimize the local side effects that occur with inhaled steroid administration?

a. _____

b. _____

c. _____

## CLINICAL APPLICATION

*Identify each of the following statements as either true or false.*

36. True or False: In asthma, a corticosteroid use is considered a controller agent rather than a relieving agent.

37. True or False: In asthma, the emphasis has shifted from the use of inhaled corticosteroids as the first line of defense to the second line of defense to reduce inflammation.

38. True or False: Asthma is now understood to be a chronic inflammatory disorder rather than a disease emphasizing bronchospasm.

39. True or False: Only moderate and severe persistent asthma should be treated with inhaled corticosteroids.

40. True or False: Inhaled steroids plus $\beta$ agonists reduce morbidity and airway hyperresponsiveness.

41. True or False: For long-term control of mild persistent asthma in children, corticosteroids represent the first line of antiinflammatory therapy.

Don't use a corticosteroid to treat an acute asthma attack. Systemic application is indicated here.

42. Remember why?

For those with inadequate symptom control a long-term $\beta_2$ agonist can be used.

43. Remember why?

44. In asthma, to verify peak expiratory flow rate a _____ _____

_____ should be used.

## Use of Corticosteroids in Chronic Obstructive Pulmonary Disease

45. What is the different pattern of inflammatory cells between chronic obstructive pulmonary disease (COPD) and asthma?

46. True or False: Unlike for asthma, oral or parenteral steroids are often given for acute exacerbation of COPD.

## NATIONAL BOARD OF RESPIRATORY CARE–TYPE QUESTIONS

1. Corticosteroids are naturally secreted by which of the following?
   a. Thymal cortex: outer zone
   b. Adrenal cortex: outer zone
   c. Adrenal cortex: inner zone
   d. Thymal cortex: inner zone

2. Which of the following are clinical indicators for intranasal aerosol steroids?
   I. Seasonal allergies
   II. Acute persistent mild asthma
   III. Perennial allergies
   IV. Acute exacerbation of COPD
      a. I and III only
      b. II and IV only
      c. I, II, and III only
      d. I, II, III, and IV

3. Corticosteroids are described as which of the following?
   a. Bronchodilators
   b. Smooth muscle dilators
   c. Antiinflammatory
   d. Lipid soluble

4. Which of the following occur during an asthma attack?
   I. Bronchospasm
   II. Release of epinephrine
   III. Mucosal edema
   IV. Increased secretions
      a. I, II, III, and IV
      b. I, II, and III only
      c. I, III, and IV only
      d. II, III, and IV only

5. Fluticasone propionate and salmeterol are drugs that are found in:
   a. Azmacort
   b. Advair Diskus
   c. Symbicort
   d. QVAR

6. Which of the following represents an advantage of local over systemic administration of corticosteroids?
   a. Greater systemic side effects
   b. Higher dose required
   c. Direct acting
   d. No side effects

7. Allergic and nonallergic rhinitis would be treated with which of the following forms of corticosteroid?
   a. Pill
   b. Nasal spray
   c. Aerosol
   d. Injection

8. All but which of the following are side effects seen with systemic administration of corticosteroids?
   a. HPA suppression
   b. Growth retardation
   c. Diuresis
   d. Osteoporosis

9. Which of the following describes aerosol administration of corticosteroids?
   a. It is associated with no side effects.
   b. It produces severe side effects.
   c. It results in more systemic than local side effects.
   d. It results in more local than systemic side effects.

10. Which of the following minimizes local side effects associated with use of inhaled corticosteroids?
   a. Use of a spacer device
   b. Rinsing the mouth after each treatment
   c. Taking the lowest dose possible
   d. All the above

11. One of the primary reasons for using aerosolized glucocorticoids is to minimize _____ suppression.
   a. Eosinophil
   b. Neutrophil
   c. Adrenal
   d. White blood cell

**118**

12. Which of the following is/are the most common inflammatory lung disease(s)?
    I. Bronchiolitis
    II. Emphysema
    III. Asthma
    IV. Chronic bronchitis
        a. I and II only
        b. III and IV only
        c. I, III, and IV only
        d. I, II, and III only

13. Early asthmatic response is caused by:
    a. Eosinophils
    b. Neutrophils
    c. Plasma leakage
    d. IgE

14. A bolus of steroid has been given to an adult asthmatic who is doing poorly. The bolus will help to:
    a. Restore β-agonist responsiveness
    b. Reduce eosinophils
    c. Increase white blood cells
    d. Decrease plasma leakage

15. The common side effects of inhaled steroids include:
    I. Oral thrush
    II. Excessive oral secretions
    III. Dysphonia
    IV. Yellowing of the teeth
        a. I and IV only
        b. I and III only
        c. I, II, and III only
        d. I, II, III, and IV

16. What is the benefit of using Pulmicort Respules as compared with the Pulmicort Turbuhaler?
    a. Less drug is being delivered
    b. Greater bronchodilator response
    c. Fewer side effects
    d. Other bronchodilators can be added

17. Symbicort is a combination of:
    a. Albuterol and fluticasone
    b. Budesonide and formoterol
    c. Atrovent and fluticasone
    d. Budesonide and salmeterol

18. If a drug such as flunisolide shows a peak plasma level quickly, within 2 minutes, this would indicate:
    a. Reduced removal from the body by the kidney
    b. Excessive dose delivery
    c. Excessive oropharyngeal deposition
    d. Good absorption by the lung

19. Cells that are inhibited and are involved in airway inflammation do *not* include:
    a. Macrophages
    b. Eosinophils
    c. Mast cells
    d. Epithelial cells

Mrs. Peacock has been prescribed triamcinolone acetonide (Azmacort) 100 µg/puff (2 puffs qid), as treatment for moderate asthma.

1. How much triamcinolone will she receive in a 24-hour period?

Mrs. Peacock has never used an MDI with a spacer device.

2. When instructing her in the use of her MDI, what points must you cover?

    a. _____

    b. _____

    c. _____

    d. _____

(Appendix D in the textbook has the current NAEPP guidelines.)

Betty is a 29-year-old with asthma, and lives in Atlanta. It is springtime, so the pollen is extremely thick. She monitors herself and is considered at present to require step 1 care in her management of asthma. When she has minor exacerbations she uses her MDI albuterol. Over the past 2 weeks she has had several more exacerbations. Her symptoms include night-time coughing, increased wheezing, and tightness in her chest, and her peak expiratory flow rate (PEFR) has dropped 22%. She has come to the doctor's office and the asthma educator sees her.

1. What should the educator recommend to Betty?

Betty has agreed to this change. It is now 4 days later and she is not getting better. In fact, her night-time symptoms are worse and she is not able to sleep through the night because of her coughing. She calls the asthma educator, seeking advice.

2. What is the next recommendation for Betty?

(Appendix D has the current Global Initiative for Chronic Obstructive Lung Disease [GOLD] guidelines.)

Andy is a 69-year-old with bronchiectasis. He is in the emergency department with complaints of increasing shortness of breath, chest tightness, and increased coughing with increased sputum production. His sputum is more purulent in appearance and he has a fever. His respiratory rate is 34 breaths/min and his $SpO_2$ is 90%. He is taking albuterol by MDI at home. He states that he tried to use his MDI but without success, because he was too short of breath.

1. What immediate therapy should be administered? List four options.

   a. _____

   b. _____

   c. _____

   d. _____

2. What are three symptoms this patient exhibits that indicate the need for antibiotics?

   a. _____

   b. _____

3. In COPD patients with infections, what are two predominant bacteria recovered from patients with exacerbation of COPD?

   a. _____

   b. _____

4. For what reason(s) did Andy have an exacerbation of his COPD?

5. When Andy is discharged, what respiratory home medications should he use to prevent future exacerbations?

   a. _____

   b. _____

6. List three respiratory care criteria used to determine when Andy is ready to be discharged.

   a. _____

   b. _____

   c. _____

# 12 Nonsteroidal Antiasthma Agents

## CHAPTER OBJECTIVES

*After answering the following questions, the reader should be able to:*

1. Discuss the indications for nonsteroidal antiasthma agents
2. List available nonsteroidal antiasthma agents used in respiratory therapy
3. Differentiate between the specific nonsteroidal antiasthma agents
4. Describe the routes of administration available for various nonsteroidal antiasthma agents
5. Describe the mode of action for various nonsteroidal antiasthma agents
6. Discuss the use of nonsteroidal antiasthma agents in the treatment of asthma

## KEY TERMS AND DEFINITIONS

*Complete the following questions by writing the answer in the space provided.*

1. Connective tissue cells that contain heparin and histamine are called _____

   _____.

2. Also known as cromolyn-like agents, these agents are used as a prophylactic to treat the inflammatory response in

   asthma: _____ _____ _____.

3. Chemical mediators that cause inflammation are called _____.

4. An agent that blocks the inflammatory response in asthma is called a(n) _____.

## CLINICAL INDICATION FOR NONSTEROIDAL ANTIASTHMA AGENTS

*Complete the following questions by writing the answer in the space provided.*

5. Alternatives to low-dose corticosteroids in step 2 asthma include _____ and

   _____.

6. In infants and children, _____ and _____ are alternatives to inhaled
   corticosteroids in step 2 asthma because of their safety profiles.

7. All the nonsteroidal antiasthma drugs described in Chapter 12 are _____, not relievers.

8. What would be an indication for the initiation of controller drug therapy?

9. The following is a list of drugs that are either controllers or relievers. Place a **C** next to the drug if it is a controller and an **R** if it is a reliever.

a. Systemic corticosteroids: _____

b. Oral corticosteroids: _____

c. Leukotriene modifiers: _____

d. Cromolyn sodium: _____

e. Nedocromil sodium: _____

f. Inhaled anticholinergic bronchodilators: _____

## MECHANISMS OF INFLAMMATION IN ASTHMA

Asthma is a chronic inflammatory disorder of the airways. Asthma can be divided into two categories: extrinsic and intrinsic. Extrinsic, or allergic, asthma is allergy based, is IgE mediated, and is associated with younger subjects. Intrinsic or nonallergic asthma shows no evidence of sensitivity to inhaled allergens, is associated with adults, and may be driven by T cells (lymphocytes) and release of cytokines.

The inflammatory process is complex and incompletely understood. Release of mediators and enzymes from many cell types, including mast cells that release leukotrienes, are a result of specific (antigens) and nonspecific (e.g., dust) stimuli. Nerve fibers of the noncholinergic nonadrenergic system release mediators that contribute to local inflammatory effects. Nitric oxide release also may contribute to epithelial cell damage. Improved understanding of the inflammatory process has increased interest in developing drugs targeted at interrupting the inflammatory process.

10. List three components of asthma:

a. _____

b. _____

c. _____

## CROMOLYN-LIKE (MAST CELL–STABILIZING) AGENTS

### Cromolyn Sodium (Disodium Cromoglycate)

Cromolyn sodium (Intal) is an inhaled prophylactic, antiallergenic, antiasthmatic drug that has no bronchodilating capability. It is a nonsteroidal antiinflammatory agent that helps to stabilize the mast cell. Intal is available in metered dose inhaler (MDI) form and as a nebulizer solution. Intal is recommended for use in mild to moderate asthma.

Asthma has an early phase and a late phase. The early-phase response is bronchospasm, peaking in 15 minutes and declining over the next hour. It may be self-limiting; however, progression of other cellular events continues. The late asthmatic phase is the result of the release of inflammatory mediators. It occurs 6 to 8 hours after a challenge and may last for 24 hours. Intal is effective in blocking mast cell degranulation, the late-phase reaction.

Intal has shown success when used for both allergic and nonallergic asthma and exercised-induced asthma. Cromolyn is a safe drug with a high therapeutic margin and minimal side effects. Cromolyn has several uses besides that of an antiasthmatic. It is used as a nasal spray (Nasalcrom) for allergic rhinitis. It also has been used as a cough inhibitor for patients receiving angiotensin-converting-enzyme (ACE) inhibitors and as an effective agent for decreasing sickling in sickle cell disease.

Used occasionally, Intal will give protection in 15 minutes when taken before exercise and in 30 minutes before exposure to a specific antigen such as cat dander. For seasonal allergy, Intal should be started at least 1 week before exposure. Continual use of cromolyn is indicated for some patients and may allow decreased dosing with steroids and bronchodilators.

11. The brand name for cromolyn sodium is _____.

12. The 1% nebulizer solution contains _____ mg in 2 ml of aqueous solution.

13. As compared with the nebulizer solution, the MDI administers _____ mg per dose.

14. List three modes of action of cromolyn sodium:

 a. _____

 b. _____

 c. _____

15. It may take _____ to _____ weeks of cromolyn sodium use before reducing the concomitant therapy of bronchodilator or steroid use.

16. True or False: Cromolyn sodium has no bronchodilating action and should not be used during acute bronchospasm.

Really, cromolyn sodium is fairly safe. Only 2% of patients experience side effects, and these side effects aren't that bad. The nebulized solution may produce the following side effects: cough, nasal congestion wheezing, sneezing, and nasal itching.

### Nedocromil Sodium (Tilade)

Nedocromil sodium (Tilade) is a prophylactic antiasthmatic agent in an MDI formulation. It is a second-generation cromolyn-like drug, which has no bronchodilator properties. Control of mild persistent asthma symptoms requires regular use. Nedocromil is an antiinflammatory controller drug that inhibits the activity of multiple inflammatory cells including mast cells, eosinophils, epithelial cells, and sensory neurons. The drug is well tolerated, with unpleasant taste being the most common complaint and to a lesser extent headache and nausea.

17. Like cromolyn, nedocromil sodium is not a reliever but a _____; it has no

_____ properties and is not indicated for _____ bronchospasm.

18. The recommended dosage by MDI for maintenance therapy in asthma is 2 inhalations, 4 times per day; this would

 give _____ mg of drug per day.

Clinical efficacy of nedocromil sodium: In adults improvement was greatest in mild to moderate asthma and when used with bronchodilator therapy. In children there seems to be significant improvement in peak flow rates and a decrease in use of bronchodilators. As a bonus, 4 mg bid has been shown to be as effective as 5 mg of cromolyn sodium qid.

### ANTILEUKOTRIENE AGENTS

The leukotrienes are members of a group of biologically active fatty acids and are lipid mediators of inflammation. They are not stored in cells but are synthesized after an appropriate stimulus including antigen challenge and cytokine exposure. Each of the following cell types has the ability to synthesize leukotrienes: eosinophils, mast cells, monocytes, macrophages, basophils, neutrophils, and lymphocytes. The leukotrienes bind to specific leukotriene receptors to exert their effects.

19. Name three antileukotriene agents that have been approved for use:

 a. _____

 b. _____

 c. _____

20. What is the indication for antileukotriene agents?

21. Zyflo is approved for children _____ years of age and older.

*Complete the following questions about zileuton (Zyflo) by writing the answer in the space provided.*

22. The recommended dosage for asthma is _____.

23. One tablet should be taken at each _____ and at _____.

24. _____ _____ _____ should be evaluated periodically during treatment.

25. Two drugs that zileuton interacts with are _____ and _____.

*Complete the following questions about zafirlukast (Accolate) by writing the answer in the space provided.*

26. Accolate has been approved for children aged _____ years and older.

27. This drug inhibits asthma reactions induced by _____, cold air, _____, and aspirin.

28. Children 5–11 years of age take an oral _____-mg tablet bid; for children 12 years of age

and older an oral _____-mg tablet bid is available.

29. Instruct the child to take the drug _____ hour before eating or _____ hours after eating, because food reduces mean bioavailability.

*Complete the following questions about montelukast (Singulair) by writing the answer in the space provided.*

30. Singulair is the one antileukotriene agent that has been approved for children under the age of

_____ years.

31. Singulair is available in _____ and _____ form and can be taken with or without meals.

32. Metabolism is accomplished primarily by the _____.

The antileukotrienes are particularly useful in controlling exercise-induced, aspirin-induced, and, to a lesser extent, allergy-induced asthma. They are indicated for use in the management of chronic asthma, ranging from mild to severe. Use of antileukotrienes as a combination therapy with other asthma drugs has resulted in a decreased need for β agonists and steroids in some patients. Approximately 50% to 70% of patients have a clinical response to antileukotrienes. Steroids are the most effective antiinflammatory agents, and have a broad range of activity. Antileukotrienes affect only one biochemical pathway, thus they have limited antiinflammatory activity. The antileukotrienes are the newest class of drugs approved for treatment of asthma. Although they appear to be safe, it will be important to monitor their use. Review Table 12-2 in the textbook for comparative features of the currently available antileukotriene agents. Box 12-3 in the textbook lists advantages and disadvantages of antileukotriene drug therapy in managing asthma.

33. A combination of _____ and _____ results in greater lung function than when each of these drugs is taken separately.

## MONOCLONAL ANTIBODIES

The newest nonsteroidal agent used to treat asthma is a monoclonal antibody called omalizumab.

34. Briefly describe the mode of action of omalizumab (Xolair).

*Identify the following questions about omalizumab (Xolair) as either true or false.*

35. True or False: Xolair is not a replacement for corticosteroids.

36. True or False: Xolair is a controller, not a reliever, for uncontrolled moderate to severe persistent asthma.

37. True or False: There may be a need to increase asthma rescue agents with the use of Xolair.

## NATIONAL BOARD OF RESPIRATORY CARE–TYPE QUESTIONS

Now that you've had a chance to review this material, try doing these NBRC-type questions. When you're finished, compare your responses with the answer key at the end of the book.

1. If a patient experiences an asthma attack as a result of exposure to cats, the asthma would be categorized as which of the following?
   a. Intrinsic
   b. Extrinsic
   c. Autoimmune
   d. Intangible

2. All but which of the following occurs during as asthma attack?
   a. Bronchospasm
   b. Mucosal edema
   c. Increased secretion production
   d. Cilia hyperactivity

3. Concerning cytokines, which of the following is true?
   a. They are released by B lymphocytes.
   b. They cause sloughing and death of eosinophils.
   c. They cause accumulation of eosinophils.
   d. Both a and b

4. The increase and activation of eosinophils are associated with which of the following?
   a. Preasthma attack
   b. Increased airway inflammation
   c. Lessened asthma severity
   d. Decreased production of leukotrienes

5. Cromolyn sodium is classified as which of the following?
   a. Bronchodilator
   b. Cholinergic
   c. Corticosteroid
   d. Antiasthmatic

6. Cromolyn sodium is indicated for all but which of the following conditions?
   a. Acute asthma
   b. Asthma prophylaxis
   c. Exercise-induced bronchoconstriction (EIB)
   d. Allergic rhinitis

7. Cromolyn sodium accomplishes which of the following?
   I. Stabilizes leukotrienes
   II. Stabilizes mast cells
   III. Prevents histamine release
   IV. Prevents eosinophil degranulation
      a. I and III only
      b. I and IV only
      c. II and III only
      d. II and IV only

8. In infants and children, which of the following drugs are alternatives to inhaled corticosteroids?
   I. Cromolyn sodium
   II. Nedocromil sodium
   III. Beclomethasone
   IV. Salmeterol
      a. I and II only
      b. II and III only
      c. I, II, and IV only
      d. I, II, III, and IV

9. All of the following drugs are considered to be controllers for asthma *except:*
   a. Oral corticosteroids
   b. Leukotriene modifiers
   c. Systemic corticosteroids
   d. Nedocromil sodium

10. All of the following represent modes of action of cromolyn sodium *except:*
    a. Antiasthmatic
    b. Antiallergic
    c. Mast cell stabilizer
    d. Bronchial smooth muscle relaxer

11. Which of the following is *not* a true statement concerning nedocromil sodium?
    a. It relaxes vascular smooth muscle.
    b. It has no bronchodilating effects.
    c. It is a controller.
    d. It is not for use in acute bronchospasm.

12. The antileukotriene modifier that is approved for children less than 5 years of age is:
    a. Zyflo
    b. Singulair
    c. Accolate
    d. Xolair

13. Which of the following is an indication for antileukotrienes?
    a. Relaxation of bronchial smooth muscle through metabolic pathways
    b. Chronic treatment of asthma
    c. Acute severe bronchospasm
    d. Acute moderate bronchospasm

14. Drugs that interact with Zyflo and may require dosing adjustment of Zyflo include:
    I. Theophylline
    II. Beclomethasone
    III. Cromolyn sodium
    IV. Warfarin
        a. I and IV only
        b. II and III only
        c. I and II only
        d. II and IV only

15. For treatment of chronic asthma a combination of _____ and _____
    results in greater lung function than when these drugs are taken separately.
    a. $\beta_2$ Agonist and steroid
    b. $\beta_2$ Agonist and cromolyn sodium
    c. Corticosteroid and antileukotriene
    d. $\beta_2$ Agonist and antileukotriene

Your patient, Bruce Jenkins, is a world class decathlete who suffers from exercise-induced bronchospasm (EIB). His physician has prescribed a β agonist to treat his bronchospasm and has asked for your recommendation as to which antiasthmatic to try.

1. What do you recommend? Why?

2. What delivery device do you recommend for Bruce?

3. Bruce is concerned about how much medication to take and when he should take the medication so as not to have bronchospasm. What would you tell him?

4. Bruce forgets his cromolyn sodium before exercise one day and experiences some mild bronchospasm. What should he do?

# 13 Aerosolized Antiinfective Agents

## CHAPTER OBJECTIVES

*After answering the following questions, the reader should be able to:*

1. Discuss the indications for inhaled antiinfective agents
2. List all available inhaled antiinfective agents used in respiratory therapy
3. Differentiate between the specific antiinfective agent formulations
4. Discuss the route of administration available for the various antiinfective agents
5. Describe the mode of action for the various antiinfective agents
6. Recognize side effects for the various antiinfective agents
7. Discuss the use of each antiinfective agent in the treatment of lung disease

## KEY TERMS AND DEFINITIONS

*Complete the following questions by writing the answer in the space provided.*

1. An agent that stops a virus from replicating is called _____.

2. The virus that causes formation of syncytial masses in infected cell structures is _____

   _____ _____.

3. An inherited disease of the exocrine glands, affecting several organs including the lung, and characterized by

   thickened secretions and respiratory infections, is called _____ _____.

4. An interstitial plasma cell pneumonia caused by the organism *Pneumocystis carinii (jiroveci)* is

   _____ _____ _____. The pneumonia is common
   among patients with lowered immune system response.

5. An agent that kills a virus is described as _____.

6. A _____ can be defined as an obligate intracellular parasite, containing either DNA or RNA
   that reproduces by synthesis of subunits within the host cell and causing disease as a consequence of this replication.

## CLINICAL INDICATIONS FOR AEROSOLIZED ANTIINFECTIVE AGENTS

7. What is the indication for the following aerosolized antiinfective agents? Also give the brand name. (*Hint:* Review
   Table 13-1 in the textbook.)

   a. Pentamidine isethionate: _____, _____

   b. Ribavirin: _____, _____

   c. Tobramycin: _____, _____

   d. Zanamivir: _____, _____

**131**

## Introduction of Aerosolized Pentamidine (NebuPent)

Pentamidine isethionate (NebuPent) is an antiprotozoal agent. It is effective for use as a prophylactic and for acute episodes of *Pneumocystis carinii* (also known as *pneumocystis jiroveci*) infection. *Pneumocystis carinii* is the causative organism for *Pneumocystis* pneumonia (PCP). PCP is an opportunistic infection in subjects with acquired immune deficiency syndrome (AIDS) and in others who are immunocompromised. Pentamidine can be administered as an aerosol or given parenterally. As with other aerosolized medications, the inhalation route offers direct organ targeting with higher concentration of the drug and fewer systemic side effects. In AIDS subjects the normal treatment dose is 300 mg via inhalation once every 4 weeks. The drug is supplied as a powder that must be reconstituted with sterile water, not saline. Use of a nebulizer that can produce a mass median diameter (MMD) of 1 to 2 μm is required. This helps prevent production of large particles that deposit and irritate the large airways and allows the smaller, appropriately sized particles to reach the lung periphery.

The exact mode of action of pentamidine is unknown, although it may have multiple effects. Resistance to pentamidine by *P. carinii* has not been shown. Systemic administration of pentamidine is effective against PCP, but more than 50% of patients experience adverse side effects. It was because of the severe side effects that aerosol administration was investigated. Side effects with aerosolized pentamidine involve both local airway effects and systemic side effects. Pulmonary effects include cough, shortness of breath, bad taste, bronchospasm, and spontaneous pneumothorax. Systemic side effects include conjunctivitis, rash, neutropenia, pancreatitis, renal insufficiency, hypoglycemia, diabetes, digital necrosis of the feet, and extrapulmonary *P. carinii* infection. Chronic treatment with aerosolized pentamidine can lead to significant systemic absorption and the same side effects as seen with parenteral administration. Use of a bronchodilator before inhalation of pentamidine can reduce the local side effects. Pentamidine is not known to be teratogenic (causing fetal deformities), mutagenic, or carcinogenic. However, there are concerns regarding environmental exposure. Exposure to the aerosolized drug has been reported to cause bronchospasm and conjunctivitis in health care workers. There also is a risk of tuberculosis (TB) transmission when treating patients with acquired immunodeficiency syndrome (AIDS) because of the close association of TB and AIDS. Because of this, precautionary measures are suggested when administering aerosolized pentamidine.

8. What is the name of the nebulizer system recommended for use with pentamidine administration?

9. What is the difference between the Respirgard II nebulizer system and a simple, small volume nebulizer? (*Hint:* See Figure 13-3 in the textbook.)

10. For effective nebulization of pentamidine the mass median diameter of particles should be in the range of

_____  _____ μm.

11. True or False: It is recommended that administration of pentamidine take place in a negative-flow (pressure) room or in an isolation booth.

12. The most common local side effect from aerosol administration of pentamidine is a(n) _____.

## RIBAVIRIN

Ribavirin is an antiviral, active against respiratory syncytial virus (RSV), herpes simplex virus, and influenza virus. It's virostatic, not virucidal, so it only inhibits DNA and RNA viruses. When it is given by aerosol, drug levels are greater in the sputum than in the blood stream. Again, ribavirin is indicated for hospitalized infants and young children with severe lower respiratory tract infections caused by RSV, which will result in bronchiolitis or pneumonia; all patients receiving mechanical ventilation because of RSV; and infants and children at serious risk for developing severe lower respiratory tract disease.

Ribavirin is administered by a large-volume nebulizer system known as the SPAG-2 (small particle aerosol generator). The treatment drug dose is 20 mg/ml and length of time for administration is 12 to 18 hours per day for 3 to 7 days. The MMD of particles from the SPAG-2 is in the range of 1.3 μm. Nebulized medications can be delivered into a hood, tent, or mechanical ventilator circuit for intubated patients. Drug delivery with mechanical ventilators is not recommended because of the risk of ventilator malfunction, but this has been successfully and safely carried out. Filters on the expiratory side of the patient circuit are a must in order to prevent malfunction of the expiratory valve from drug precipitate. Respiratory therapists should consistently monitor these filters and the function of the expiratory valve of the ventilator. During treatment these filters must be changed regularly to prevent increased resistance to exhalation by the patient.

13. What is the dose of ribavirin administered by the SPAG-2 nebulizer system?

14. When using a SPAG-2 nebulizer system in-line with a mechanical ventilator, what should the respiratory therapist consistently monitor?

15. What is the reason for near continuous nebulization of ribavirin?

Side effects of aerosolized ribavirin include deterioration of pulmonary function, pneumothorax, apnea, bacterial pneumonia, cardiovascular instability, and reticulocytosis. Rash, eyelid erythema, and conjunctivitis also have been reported. The more common side effects include skin irritation and decrease in pulmonary function; and equipment malfunction due to drug precipitate occurs.

Environmental exposure to ribavirin is a concern. The drug is mutagenic, carcinogenic, teratogenic, and embryocidal in animal species. Health care workers have reported effects such as conjunctivitis, headache, rhinitis, nausea, rash, dizziness, pharyngitis, lacrimation, bronchospasm, and chest pain. Environmental containment and a scavenger system should be used; these are superior to personal protective barriers. Pregnant women should not be in the treatment area.

16. List three common side effects of ribavirin:

a. _____

b. _____

c. _____

### RESPIRATORY SYNCYTIAL VIRUS IMMUNE GLOBULIN INTRAVENOUS (HUMAN)-RESPIGAM

What is RSV immune globulin intravenous (human)? It's a neutralizing antibody to RSV and is available as RespiGam. RSV-IGIV is indicated to prevent serious lower respiratory tract infections in children younger than 2 years with bronchopulmonary dysplasia (BPD) or a history of premature birth.

17. RSV-IGIV is indicated for two different groups of children:

a. _____

b. _____

18. How is RSV-IGIV delivered? (*Hint:* What do you think the IV stands for?)

19. High-risk children are given the drug during the RSV season, which runs from _____

_____ in the northern hemisphere.

## PALIVIZUMAB (SYNAGIS)

20. Palivizumab (Synagis) has been approved for the prevention and treatment of RSV in _____
infants and those with bronchopulmonary dysplasia, and children with congenital heart disease.

21. It is given by _____ injection once a month during RSV season.

## AEROSOLIZED TOBRAMYCIN

Cystic fibrosis (CF) is one disease state in which nebulized antibiotics have been used. Lungs of CF patients are chronically infected with *Pseudomonas aeruginosa,* a gram-negative microbe, and *Staphylococcus aureus,* a gram-positive microbe. Most antibiotics effective against *P. aeruginosa* are ineffective when taken orally, which means IV or aerosolized administration must be considered.

Tobramycin (TOBI) is an antibiotic effective against gram-negative infections and has a bactericidal effect. TOBI is formulated as a nebulizer solution with 300 mg in a 5-ml ampoule. Dosage is 300 mg q12h for 28 days. After 28 days without TOBI treatment, the cycle repeats. It is recommended that TOBI be administered with the PARI LC Plus and DeVilbiss Pulmo-Aide compressor. TOBI has been recommended for use in managing chronic infection to treat and prevent early colonization with *P. aeruginosa* in CF and to help maintain present lung function or to reduce the rate of deterioration. Tobramycin has been shown to have a high drug level in bronchial secretions and a low blood level. Administration of TOBI should follow other normal pulmonary treatments, and tobramycin should not be mixed with dornase alfa in the same nebulizer treatment. TOBI can be used in individuals 6 years of age or older. Although some clinically significant side effects can be seen with parenteral administration of tobramycin (see Box 13-10 in the textbook), only a few side effects are seen with inhalation of TOBI. These include voice alteration and tinnitus (a subjective noise sensation often described as ringing in the ears). Local airway irritation resulting in cough and bronchospasm may occur. Evaluate these changes by peak flow rate measurement and breath sounds. Research data have shown that use of TOBI results in improved lung function, reduced hospitalizations, and reduced use of IV antipseudomonal antibiotics. Significant drug resistance has not been observed.

22. Why should TOBI be used with patients diagnosed with cystic fibrosis?

a. _____

b. _____

23. True or False: TOBI should be taken before other therapies, including chest physiotherapy and bronchodilator therapy, in order to achieve the greatest airway clearance of secretions.

24. True or False: TOBI can be mixed with dornase alfa to achieve a synergistic effect.

25. Is there a specific nebulizer and compressor that is recommended for delivery of TOBI? If yes, what is it?

26. True or False: Local airway irritation resulting in bronchospasm can be evaluated by listening to breath sounds.

27. If an injectable antibiotic is nebulized, a flow rate ranging from _____to

_____ L/min is recommended because of the viscosity of antibiotic solutions.

## INHALED ZANAMIVIR

Zanamivir (Relenza) is an antiviral agent approved for use in the treatment of influenza in adults and children more than 5 years of age within the first 2 days of infection. Zanamivir is available in a dry powder inhaler (DPI). Each blister contains 5 mg of drug. The treatment dose is 10 mg (two inhalations of 5 mg each) bid (q12 h) for 5 days. Inhaled zanamivir has been shown to decrease the duration of influenza symptoms when treatment is started within 2 days of onset of symptoms. Zanamivir is not approved for influenza prophylaxis, but some data suggest it may provide some prophylactic benefit.

Some adverse side effects have been reported with the use of zanamivir. Bronchospasm has been reported in asthma and chronic obstructive pulmonary disease (COPD) patients, along with decreased expiratory flow rates. Drug treatment should be suspended if bronchospasm or decreased pulmonary function occurs. *Note:* Bacterial lung infections may mimic influenza. Inappropriate treatment with zanamivir in bacterial infections, noninfluenza viral infections, or in patients with an exacerbation of COPD, can lead to serious complications. Zanamivir provides no benefit for patients who are not infected with influenza virus. Because of the lack of a clinically easy and inexpensive diagnostic test to confirm the presence of influenza infection, inappropriate use places some patients at risk and contributes to increased costs. Patients also should be monitored for allergic reactions.

28. Each blister of zanamivir contains _____ mg of drug and the patient should have a total

treatment dose of _____ mg.

29. True or False: Zanamivir can be used for patients who are not infected with influenza virus.

## RESPIRATORY CARE ASSESSMENT OF AEROSOLIZED ANTIINFECTIVE AGENTS

*Identify each of the following statements as either true or false.*

30. True or False: A short-acting β agonist can be given to prevent coughing and bronchospasm with administration of pentamidine.

31. True or False: When administering ribavirin to a child receiving mechanical ventilation, the respiratory therapist should consistently monitor in-line filters for obstruction due to drug precipitate.

32. True or False: Mouth rinsing should be done after administration of aerosolized TOBI.

33. True or False: A patient using zanamivir DPI should not use a bronchodilator if airway irritation causes bronchospasm.

## NATIONAL BOARD OF RESPIRATORY CARE–TYPE QUESTIONS

Try to answer the following NBRC-type questions.

1. Pentamidine is considered to be which of the following?
   a. Antifungal
   b. Antiparasitic
   c. Antiprotozoal
   d. Antibacterial

2. Pentamidine may be administered via which of the following route(s) of administration?
   a. Oral
   b. Inhalation
   c. IV
   d. Both b and c

3. The only device currently approved by the U.S. Food and Drug Administration for the administration of pentamidine (NebuPent) is which of the following:
   a. SPAG-2
   b. Respirgard II
   c. AeroTech II
   d. Fisoneb

4. Small volume nebulizers (SVNs) used to deliver pentamidine should be equipped with which of the following?
   I. Inspiratory filter
   II. Expiratory filter
   III. One-way valves
   IV. Compression generators
      a. III and IV only
      b. II and III only
      c. I and II only
      d. I, II, and IV only

5. Ribavirin is classified as which of the following?
   a. Antiprotozoal
   b. Antifungal
   c. Antibacterial
   d. Antiviral

6. Which of the following is the clinical indication for ribavirin?
   a. Prophylactic treatment of PCP
   b. Treatment of RSV infection
   c. Treatment of chronic *Pseudomonas aeruginosa* infection
   d. Treatment of noninfluenza virus infection

7. For effective nebulization of pentamidine the mass median diameter of particles should be in the range of:
   a. 1 to 2 μm
   b. 3 to 4 μm
   c. 5 to 8 μm
   d. 1 to 10 μm

8. The standard dose of ribavirin administered by the SPAG-2 nebulizer system is:
   a. 10 mg/ml
   b. 20 mg/ml
   c. 30 mg/ml
   d. 35 mg/ml

9. In the northern hemisphere RSV season runs from:
   a. January to April
   b. January to November
   c. November to April
   d. December and January

10. Which of the following is *not* an indication for TOBI use in cystic fibrosis patients?
    a. To treat influenza type B infections
    b. To treat and prevent early colonization of *P. aeruginosa*
    c. To maintain present lung function
    d. To reduce the rate of deterioration of lung function

11. Which of the following nebulizers is recommended for use to administer TOBI?
    a. SPAG-2
    b. Respirgard II
    c. Aerojet III
    d. PARI-LC Plus

12. Which of the following are indications for RSV-IGIV (RespiGam)?
    I. Children with BPD and who are less than 2 years of age
    II. Children less than 2 years old and who have a history of premature birth
    III. Children less than 2 years old and diagnosed with cystic fibrosis
    IV. Children less than 6 months old, with BPD without influenza virus
        a. I and II only
        b. I and III only
        c. II and IV only
        d. I, II, and IV only

13. Which of the following statements is *true* regarding TOBI?
    a. Chest physiotherapy should be administered as the patient is breathing TOBI.
    b. Dornase alfa may be mixed with TOBI to achieve a synergistic effect.
    c. TOBI should be administered after administration of all other therapy or medications.
    d. TOBI should be mixed with a short-acting β-agonist to prevent bronchospasm.

14. A treatment dose of _____ mg of zanamivir is recommended for influenza infection.
    a. 5
    b. 10
    c. 20
    d. 200

15. Which of the following is the reason why ribavirin is administered for 12 to 18 hours per day for the treatment of RSV?
    a. A large quantity of drug rainout occurs because of the large particles formed from the SPAG-II device.
    b. The powder creates increased rainout of the drug within the SPAG-II nebulizer system.
    c. The drug has a short half-life in respiratory secretions.
    d. The liver metabolizes the drug quickly.

Your patient, who has been positive for human immunodeficiency virus (HIV) since 1994, presents with a CD4+ cell count of $100/mm^3$, fever, shaking, chills, and productive cough. He has had PCP once before this admission. His diagnosis is PCP, and his physician has ordered pentamidine isethionate (NebuPent) treatments qid to treat it. As you do your pretreatment assessment, the patient tells you that he has previously been given pentamidine and that "It makes me cough pretty much throughout the whole treatment."

1.  What do you recommend?

As a favor to you, one of your colleagues begins this treatment, using a small volume nebulizer.

2.  Should your colleague be using an SVN to administer pentamidine?

3.  Other than using the Respirgard II, what precautions should you take to minimize your exposure to the pentamidine?

    a.  _____

    b.  _____

    c.  _____

    d.  _____

    e.  _____

4.  What adverse effects are you likeliest to suffer as a result of exposure to pentamidine?

# 14 Antimicrobial Agents

## CHAPTER OBJECTIVES

*After answering the following questions, the reader should be able to:*

1. Define *antibiotic*
2. Describe the process involved in bacterial susceptibility testing
3. Discuss possible outcomes of antimicrobial combinations
4. List the various classes of the penicillins
5. List the various classes of the cephalosporins
6. Recognize similarities between members of the macrolides
7. Recognize similarities between members of the quinolones
8. List four mechanisms of action of antibacterials
9. List five commonly used antimycobacterials
10. Describe the commonly used azole antifungals and how they differ in spectrum of activity
11. Discuss similarities between members of the echinocandins

## KEY TERMS AND DEFINITIONS

*Complete the following by writing the answer in the space provided.*

1. Both natural and synthetic compounds that either inhibit or kill microorganisms are called _____.

2. The term _____ describes when the combined effect of two antimicrobials is greater than their added effects.

3. Natural compounds, produced by microorganisms and that either inhibit or kill other microorganisms, are called

   _____.

4. The term _____ describes when the effect of a combination of two antimicrobials is lower than the effect expected from either agent alone.

## PRINCIPLES OF ANTIMICROBIAL THERAPY

Several factors must be considered before choosing an antimicrobial agent. These include:
- Identification of the pathogen
- Determining antimicrobial susceptibility
- Consideration of host factors
- Consideration of drug factors

Each of these is discussed in the following sections.

### Identification of the Pathogen

Identification of the pathogen is the first step. This is accomplished by collecting some of the infected material for culture. The simplest and most common identification method is the Gram stain. The Gram stain separates bacteria into gram-positive strains, which stain purple, and gram-negative strains, which stain pink. Structural components in the cell walls are responsible for the difference in staining. These components determine the microbe's susceptibility to antimicrobials. The exact species of microbe is not always identified from cultures. In such cases, empirical treatment (i.e., treatment judged on the basis of experience and research most likely to be effective) is given.

5. The simplest and most common preparation by which to identify bacteria is the _____ _____.

6. Gram-positive bacteria stain _____ and gram-negative bacteria stain _____.

7. *Mycobacterium tuberculosis* requires a(n) _____-_____ stain to penetrate its waxlike cell wall.

8. Match the following common pathogens with their associated respiratory infection(s) in the adult. (*Hint:* Review Table 14-1 in the textbook for the complete listing.)

a. _____ Sinusitis

b. _____ Community-acquired pneumonia

c. _____ Hospital-acquired pneumonia

d. _____ Acute bronchitis

e. _____ Cystic fibrosis

1. *Staphylococcus aureus*
2. *Mycoplasma pneumoniae*
3. *Staphylococcus pneumoniae*
4. *Haemophilus influenzae*
5. *Streptococcus pneumoniae*
6. *Burkholderia cepacia*

## Susceptibility Testing and Resistance

The next step is a susceptibility test. A common test involves placing disks, saturated with antibiotics, on an agar plate inoculated with the microbe. If the antibiotic is effective against the microbe, no microbes will grow near the disk. This is known as the *zone of inhibition*. The larger the zone, the greater the susceptibility of the microbe. This aspect of antimicrobial therapy is critical for appropriate treatment, especially when dealing with resistant organisms. Other methods, including the elliptical test (E-test) and the broth dilution technique, can be used to obtain similar results. The minimal inhibitory concentration (MIC) of a drug and the minimal bacterial concentration (MBC) can be determined from these respective procedures.

## Host Factors

Host factors play an important role in determining appropriate drug therapy. Immunocompromised patients may fail to respond to antimicrobial therapy. Although some antimicrobials have the ability to kill microbes, an intact immune system is needed for eradication of infection. Gastric pH can affect drug absorption. Liver and kidney function play a role in drug metabolism and excretion. Organ disease may require adjustments in drug dosage. Pregnant mothers must be very careful not to take certain drugs because they may cross the placental barrier and harm the developing fetus. The teratogenic effect of many antimicrobials is not known. Some antimicrobials will selectively concentrate in certain organs or organ systems, making them more or less appropriate for use.

9. Bactericidal drugs _____ bacteria whereas bacteriostatic drugs _____ growth of bacteria.

## Pharmacodynamics and Antimicrobial Combinations

Pharmacodynamics refers to the effect a drug has on microbes as a function of concentration or time. If the microbial kill rate is proportional to drug concentration, the drug is said to have a concentration-dependent effect. If the kill rate is influenced by time, the agent is said to be time dependent. Another phenomenon exhibited by antimicrobials is the postantibiotic effect (PAE), in which bacterial growth is inhibited even after the drug level drops below detectable levels. Agents with a short PAE need to be dosed frequently.

Because microbes often are not identified precisely, empiric treatment will occasionally require the use of two or more classes of antimicrobials. These drugs should act synergistically and not antagonistically.

10. When two or more classes of antimicrobials are combined they should act _____, not antagonistically.

## MONITORING RESPONSE TO THERAPY

A response to therapy is best measured by clinical assessment of the patient. Reasons for failure can be multifocal, including inappropriate identification of microbe, inappropriate choice of agent, and inappropriate identification of host factors. Patient noncompliance also must be considered. Patients must be monitored for signs of toxicity, and if present, therapy must be adjusted appropriately.

11. Although certain laboratory parameters can be monitored to assess the efficacy of an antimicrobial regimen,

    response to therapy is best measured by _____ _____.

## ANTIBIOTICS

Alexander Fleming discovered penicillin in 1928. This discovery led to the class of antibiotics known as the β-lactams. The β-lactams include the penicillins, cephalosporins, monobactams, and carbapenems.

### Penicillins

Penicillins are widely distributed in the body and are associated with low toxicity. Most are destroyed if taken orally because of gastric pH. Ampicillin and amoxicillin are two exceptions and are stable in gastric acid. The kidney excretes penicillin, so patients with renal disease should have their drug dose decreased. Penicillins exert their effect by inhibiting cell wall synthesis and activating an autolytic system within the cell that results in self-destruction. Penicillins are bactericidal, demonstrate time-dependent killing, and act synergistically with the aminoglycosides.

The most common reaction to the penicillins is hypersensitivity. Reactions will vary from a skin rash to life-threatening anaphylaxis. Nausea, vomiting, and diarrhea are common with orally delivered penicillins.

### Cephalosporins

The cephalosporins were discovered in the 1940s. They are bactericidal, are distributed throughout the body, and have relatively few side effects. Cephalosporins inhibit cell wall synthesis, which results in cell lysis. Cephalosporins have a wide spectrum of activity, but none are effective against the enterococci. The cephalosporins can be taken orally.

They are separated into four "generations" based on their spectrum of activity. First-generation cephalosporins are generally appropriate for gram-positive infections. The second-generation agents have enhanced activity against gram-negative organisms. The third-generation cephalosporins are effective against many gram-negative infections. Cefepime is the only fourth-generation agent available in the United States. It has extended coverage against both gram-positive and gram-negative organisms.

As a group, cephalosporins are well tolerated, but their use is contraindicated in patients with a history of anaphylaxis to β-lactams. Oral drugs have produced some gastrointestinal (GI) complaints.

### Carbapenems

Carbapenems are broad-spectrum antibiotics, effective against gram-positive, gram-negative, and anaerobic bacteria. They are used for a wide variety of infectious diseases and are often reserved to treat infections caused by bacteria resistant to other agents. They are generally well tolerated, but dose adjustments are necessary in patients with decreased renal function.

### Monobactams (Aztreonam)

Aztreonam is the only commercially available agent belonging to the class of antibiotics known as the *monobactams*. Its action is similar to that of other β-lactams and is bactericidal. It is active only against gram-negative aerobic bacilli. Its use as a single agent is limited, but it has been used for urinary tract infections (UTIs) and bacteremia. Treatment is generally well tolerated.

12. Penicillins and cephalosporins exert their pharmacological activity by inhibiting _____

    _____ synthesis.

13. The only generation of cephalosporins with extended coverage of gram-positive and gram-negative organisms is

    the _____ _____.

14. Carbapenems are _____-_____ antibiotics effective against gram-positive and gram-negative bacteria.

15. True or False: The monobactam aztreonam has a mechanism of action similar to that of the other penicillins.

### Aminoglycosides

The aminoglycosides include streptomycin, gentamicin, tobramycin, netilmicin, and amikacin. They are active against gram-positive microbes and require parenteral administration. The aminoglycosides have several mechanisms of action resulting in increased cell wall permeability and lysis. They are bactericidal and exhibit concentration-dependent killing.

They are synergistic when used with β-lactams. Aminoglycosides such as gentamicin and tobramycin have been used for ventilator associated pneumonia (VAP) and as an inhaled drug (tobramycin) for cystic fibrosis (CF) patients. Nephrotoxicity and ototoxicity are the primary side effects of the aminoglycosides.

16. One example of an aminoglycoside that is used in the treatment of cystic fibrosis is _____.

17. List two aminoglycosides that are used in the treatment of ventilator-associated pneumonia (VAP):

a. _____

b. _____

## Tetracyclines

The tetracyclines are broad-spectrum antibiotics with activity against gram-positive and gram-negative strains, as well as activity against rickettsiae, chlamydiae, mycoplasmas, spirochetes, protozoa, and mycobacteria. They are available in both oral and parenteral formulations. Their action of inhibiting protein synthesis results in a bacteriostatic effect. They are used in both pulmonary and systemic infections and are effective for treatment of diseases such as Rocky Mountain spotted fever, Lyme disease, and others. They also concentrate in the skin and are useful for treatment of acne. Nausea, vomiting, and diarrhea are the most common side effects associated with the tetracyclines. However, they are contraindicated in pregnancy, during breast-feeding, and in children less than 8 years of age because they can inhibit bone growth.

18. Tetracyclines inhibit _____ _____, resulting in a bacteriostatic effect.

## Tigecycline

Tigecycline is similar in structure to the tetracycline antibiotics and is active against most gram-positive bacteria such as *Streptococcus pneumoniae* and also has activity against most gram-negative bacteria including *Haemophilus influenzae*. It is not effective against *Pseudomonas aeruginosa*. Its clinical use is for intraabdominal infections and skin infections.

## Macrolides

Macrolides, such as erythromycin, exhibit activity against gram-positive, gram-negative, and atypical bacteria, including rickettsiae, chlamydiae, and *Legionella*. Macrolides inhibit protein synthesis and are bacteriostatic in their action. Erythromycin is considered the drug of choice for the treatment of pneumonia caused by the atypical pathogens *Chlamydia pneumoniae, Mycoplasma pneumoniae*, and *Legionella pneumophila*. Erythromycin is not tolerated as well as the other macrolides, with the most common side effects being nausea, vomiting, abdominal cramps, and diarrhea. Ventricular tachycardia, dizziness, reversible hearing loss, and abnormalities in liver function have been associated with the use of macrolides. Erythromycin and clarithromycin are inhibitors of the hepatic drug metabolism cytochrome P450. Use of these macrolides with warfarin can lead to life-threatening complications.

19. The drug of choice for *Legionella* bacteria is _____.

## Telithromycin

Telithromycin is structurally related to macrolide antibiotics. It has good antimicrobial activity against respiratory pathogens that are responsible for community-acquired pneumonia (CAP) such as *S. pneumoniae, H. influenzae*, and *M. pneumoniae*.

20. A drug that has good antimicrobial activity against respiratory pathogens responsible for CAP is

_____.

## Quinolones (Fluoroquinolones)

The fluoroquinolones are widely distributed in the body, with high respiratory tract concentrations. These drugs have variable activity against gram-positive and gram-negative strains, anaerobes, atypical bacteria, and mycobacteria. Fluoroquinolones inhibit DNA synthesis, are considered bactericidal, and demonstrate concentration-dependent killing. They are effective against pulmonary tract infections, genitourinary tract infections, and skin infections. The quinolones are well tolerated and considered to be one of the safest classes of antimicrobials. However, they are not recommended for children (≤18 years of age). This is because of the results of animal studies in which immature animals have shown changes in weight-bearing joints after use of these drugs.

## Other Antibiotics

Chloramphenicol is effective against gram-positive, gram-negative, and anaerobic microbes. It distributes well into tissues, including the brain. It inhibits protein synthesis and is essentially bacteriostatic. It is highly active against *Salmonella* and rickettsial disease. Some serious side effects have occurred with the use of chloramphenicol, including aplastic anemia, gray baby syndrome in neonates, and blindness. Less toxic agents are routinely used in place of this antimicrobial.

Colistin is effective against gram-negative infections including those caused by *P. aeruginosa*. Colistin is a surface-active agent that causes disruption of bacterial cell membranes, exhibiting a bactericidal effect. Nephrotoxicity is the most serious side effect when colistin is administered intravenously. Although not approved for nebulization, colistin is routinely nebulized to patients with cystic fibrosis.

Daptomycin is active against a wide range of gram-positive bacteria and inactive against gram-negative bacteria. Daptomycin causes disruption of the cell membrane, leading to leakage of intracellular ions and rapid death. It is not indicated for treatment of pneumonia.

Trimethoprim–sulfamethoxazole (TMP–SMX) is a combination drug active against gram-positive and gram-negative microbes and against *Pneumocystis jiroveci* (formerly known as *P. carinii*). This agent blocks enzymes and ultimately prevents the synthesis of essential nucleic acids and proteins. It is bacteriostatic in action. Trimethoprim–sulfamethoxazole is tolerated fairly well, with GI symptoms and hypersensitivity being the most common side effects. Clindamycin has activity against gram-positive and anaerobic bacteria. It inhibits protein synthesis and is bacteriostatic. It distributes well into the body but has minimal penetration into the cerebrospinal fluid (CSF). It is used as an adjunct to agents with gram-negative activity in polymicrobial infections. It is used to treat anaerobic lung infections, including necrotizing pneumonia, lung abscess, empyema, aspiration pneumonia, and *Pneumocystis jiroveci* pneumonia (PCP). GI symptoms are the most common side effect.

Metronidazole has activity against protozoans and anaerobic bacteria. It is thought to break DNA strands and is bactericidal. Metronidazole penetrates well into the central nervous system (CNS) and is useful in treating brain abscess. It often is combined with other drug therapy. The most common complaints include nausea, vomiting, and a metallic taste.

Nitrofurantoin is used only for urinary tract infections because it is the only site where the concentration of this drug reaches a therapeutic level. It is bactericidal and has several mechanisms of action. Side effects of nausea and vomiting are common and can be severe enough to require discontinuation of therapy.

Vancomycin is active against gram-positive bacteria only. It prevents the formation of a rigid cell wall, resulting in cell lysis. Its bactericidal activity is useful for treatment of infections caused by methicillin-resistant *Staphylococcus aureus* (MRSA). A common reaction to rapid infusion of vancomycin is known as red man or red neck syndrome, characterized by skin itch, flushing, angioedema, and hypotension. It must be infused slowly.

Quinupristin and dalfopristin (Synercid) are synergistic agents active against gram-positive organisms and are used primarily to treat life-threatening infections caused by vancomycin-resistant *Enterococcus faecium* (VREF). Synercid inhibits protein synthesis and is bactericidal against MRSA and bacteriostatic against VREF. It must be administered through a central line as a parenteral infusion. Arthralgias (joint pain) and myalgias (muscle pain) are commonly reported side effects.

Linezolid is active against gram-positive bacteria and is indicated for the treatment of life-threatening VREF infections. It is available as an oral medication. Its most common side effects are nausea, diarrhea, and headache.

21. Vancomycin is useful for the treatment of infections caused by _____-_____

_____ _____.

## ANTIMYCOBACTERIALS

The number of tuberculosis (TB) cases has increased over the past decade in large part because of the human immunodeficiency virus (HIV) epidemic. Placing patients suspected of having TB in isolation rooms can prevent transmission of *Mycobacterium tuberculosis* by aerosolization. Patients should remain in this room until one of the three criteria listed below is met.

- They are determined not to have TB.
- They are confirmed to be noninfectious.
- They are discharged from the hospital.

Use of personal protective barriers (masks) also can help prevent transmission.

Drug treatment consists of multiple antibiotics for 6 to 12 months. Single agents should not be used because that increases the chance of development of bacterial resistance. Treatment failures are often the result of poor patient compliance with therapy and development of resistance to antibiotics. Four common drugs used to treat TB include isoniazid, rifampin, pyrazinamide, and ethambutol.

### Isoniazid

Isoniazid is absorbed when taken orally and distributed well in the body. It inhibits cell wall synthesis and is bactericidal against TB. Side effects include elevated liver enzymes. Liver function tests should be monitored, and the patient should be assessed for symptoms of hepatitis.

### Rifampin and Rifabutin

Rifampin and rifabutin, referred to as *rifamycins*, are absorbed orally with good penetration into most tissue. They are bactericidal, inhibiting the ability of bacteria to undergo cell division. Hepatotoxicity is the major side effect. It also colors body fluids a deep orange hue.

### Pyrazinamide

Pyrazinamide is an oral formulation that distributes well into most body tissues. It is bactericidal, although its mechanism of action is unknown. Nausea and vomiting are the most common side effects, but hepatic toxicity also has been reported.

### Ethambutol

Ethambutol is an oral medication that distributes well within the body. It decreases synthesis of cell wall products and is bacteriostatic. Optic neuropathy is the major toxicity associated with its use.

### Streptomycin

Streptomycin (see Aminoglycosides) is an IV formulation used as an add-on drug in patients with drug-resistant TB.

22. Drug treatment for tuberculosis consists of multiple antibiotics for _____ to

_____ months.

23. *Mycobacterium tuberculosis* is spread by _____.

## ANTIFUNGALS

The number of fungal infections has significantly increased. In part this is because of the increased number of immunocompromised patients with acquired immune deficiency syndrome (AIDS), cancer patients receiving chemotherapy, and patients undergoing organ transplantation. *Candida* species are now the fourth most commonly isolated bloodstream pathogens. Drugs used to treat fungal infections are discussed in the following sections.

### Polyenes

The polyenes include amphotericin B and nystatin. Amphotericin B has been the treatment of choice for systemic fungal infections. Nephrotoxicity has been a concern, but newer preparations of amphotericin B distribute better in the body, resulting in decreased incidence of nephrotoxicity. The polyenes increase cell permeability and are fungicidal. Amphotericin B is a first-line agent for the treatment of pulmonary fungal infections such as histoplasmosis. Rapid infusion of the drug may cause flushing, fever, and chills.

### Azoles

The systemic azoles, such as fluconazole, are available as both oral and IV formulations. Fluconazole is widely distributed in the body and is relatively nontoxic, but has a narrow spectrum of activity used for candidiasis, cryptococcal meningitis, and coccidioidomycosis. Itraconazole has a wider spectrum of activity but has greater toxicity. The azoles prevent fungal cell growth and are fungistatic. Anorexia, nausea, and vomiting are common side effects with the use of azoles.

### Echinocandins

Caspofungin, micafungin, and anidulafungin are examples of echinocandins, and they inhibit fungal cell wall synthesis. They are used to treat aspergillosis in patients when amphotericin B use is inappropriate. Common side effects include fever, rash, and thrombophlebitis.

### Flucytosine

Flucytosine is used in combination with other drugs for susceptible fungal infections such as *Candida* and *Aspergillus*. It decreases protein synthesis and is fungistatic. The most common toxic side effect is bone marrow suppression.

### Griseofulvin and Terbinafine

Griseofulvin and terbinafine are oral medications used to treat skin, hair, and nail fungi (dermatophytes). Terbinafine is well tolerated, with nausea, vomiting, and abdominal cramps being the most common side effects. Griseofulvin, however, has multiple side effects including heartburn, flatulence, inflammation of the mouth, glossodynia (tongue pain), and a black-furred tongue (a tongue coating that looks like black fur).

24. Which antifungal agent would be prescribed for a patient diagnosed with histoplasmosis?

25. Fungal infections have increased over the past years because of:

    a. _____

    b. _____

    c. _____

## ANTIVIRAL AGENTS

Each of the following agents inhibit viral replication. Nonreplicating viruses are not affected.

### Acyclovir and Valacyclovir

Acyclovir and valacyclovir (a prodrug of acyclovir) are effective against the herpesvirus family. Oral medications are generally well tolerated. A prodrug is a drug that is changed into the active agent once it is inside the body (see Chapter 6 of the textbook).

### Penciclovir and Famciclovir

Penciclovir and famciclovir, its prodrug, are similar in action to acyclovir and are well tolerated. Viral DNA synthesis and replication are affected.

### Ganciclovir and Valganciclovir

Ganciclovir and valganciclovir, its prodrug, both have activity similar to acyclovir; however, ganciclovir has much higher activity against cytomegalovirus (CMV). The most common side effect is bone marrow suppression. Ganciclovir and valganciclovir terminate viral DNA synthesis and replication.

### Cidofovir

Cidofovir (Vistide) has potent activity against a wide variety of viruses. Severe dose-dependent nephrotoxicity has been associated with the use of cidofovir. Cidofovir terminates viral replication by inhibition of viral polymerases.

### Foscarnet

Foscarnet (Foscavir) has a wide range of activity. Foscarnet works by blocking viral replication. Nephrotoxicity is a major side effect.

### Fomivirsen

Fomivirsen (Vitravene) is available only as an intravitreal (eye) preparation. Fomivirsen works by terminating viral transcription. It is used to treat cytomegalovirus (CMV) retinitis in AIDS patients.

### Amantadine and Rimantadine

Amantadine (Symadine) and rimantadine (Flumadine) are both easily absorbed from the GI tract and are well tolerated. They are used to treat influenza type A viruses. They may be used prophylactically in high-risk patients and started within 48 hours of symptoms to treat influenza type A infection. In general, amantadine and rimantadine block viral replication and viral assembly, and perhaps inhibit influenza virus from uncoating and entering of the mucosal cells of the respiratory tract.

**Oseltamivir**

Oseltamivir (Tamiflu) is a prodrug converted to oseltamivir carboxylate. It is an oral medication that inhibits influenza viruses A and B from leaving host cells to infect other cells. It is effective in the treatment of both influenza type A and B infections if started within 40 hours of symptoms. It is well tolerated, with nausea and vomiting being the side effects reported most frequently.

26. In general, antiviral agents terminate viral _____.

## NATIONAL BOARD OF RESPIRATORY CARE–TYPE QUESTIONS

Now for the NBRC-type questions!

1. The simplest and most common preparation by which to identify bacteria is the:
    a. Acid-fast stain
    b. Gram stain
    c. Ziehl–Neelsen smear
    d. Agar plate count

2. Gram-positive bacteria will stain _____, using the Gram stain method.
    a. Purple
    b. Red
    c. Pink
    d. Orange

3. An acid-fast stain is used to identify:
    a. *Pseudomonas aeruginosa*
    b. *Streptococcus pneumoniae*
    c. *Candida* species
    d. *Mycobacterium tuberculosis*

4. Which of the following common pathogens will cause community-acquired pneumonia?
    a. *Staphylococcus aureus*
    b. *Mycobacterium pneumoniae*
    c. *Pseudomonas aeruginosa*
    d. *Haemophilus influenzae*

5. A bacteriostatic drug is one that:
    a. Kills bacteria
    b. Inhibits bacterial growth
    c. Terminates replication
    d. Interferes with DNA replication

6. Although certain laboratory parameters can be monitored to assess efficacy of an antimicrobial regimen, response to therapy is best measured by:
    a. The number of antibiotics the patient is currently taking
    b. The strength of antibiotics the patient is currently taking
    c. The number of days the patient has been taking antibiotics
    d. Clinical assessment

7. Penicillins and cephalosporins exert their pharmacological activity by inhibiting:
    a. Cell wall synthesis
    b. DNA replication
    c. RNA replication
    d. Terminating viral replication

8. Broad-spectrum antibiotics are effective against:
   I. Viral infections
   II. Fungal infections
   III. Gram-positive infections
   IV. Gram-negative infections
       a. I and II only
       b. III and IV only
       c. I, II, and IV only
       d. I, II, III, and IV

9. Which of the following aminoglycosides is used to treat cystic fibrosis?
   a. Penicillin
   b. Cephalosporins
   c. Tobramycin
   d. Tetracycline

10. Which of the following drugs is used in the treatment of ventilator-associated pneumonia?
    a. Erythromycin
    b. Tetracycline
    c. Fluoroquinolones
    d. Gentamicin

11. The drug of choice for *Legionella* bacteria is:
    a. Tetracycline
    b. Erythromycin
    c. Penicillin
    d. Gentamicin

12. Methicillin-resistant *Staphylococcus aureus* (MRSA) is best treated with which of the following?
    a. Vancomycin
    b. Clindamycin
    c. Erythryomycin
    d. Gentamicin

13. A patient suspected of having TB should remain in an isolation room until which of the following criteria is met?
    a. The patient is determined not to have TB.
    b. The patient has been pharmacologically treated for 5 days.
    c. The patient has three sputum samples obtained over a 3-day period.
    d. The patient no longer needs protective barriers such as masks.

14. Drug treatment for tuberculosis consists of multiple antibiotics for:
    a. 5–7 days
    b. 12–15 days
    c. 1–2 months
    d. 6–12 months

15. A patient is diagnosed with histoplasmosis. Which of the following antifungal agents should be prescribed?
    a. Caspofungin
    b. Amphotericin B
    c. Flucytosine
    d. Rifampin

Mr. Green lives in a homeless shelter in downtown Atlanta; he moved here from New Orleans after Hurricane Katrina. He has developed symptoms including cough, production of sputum, chills, and sweating. He has come to a local hospital emergency department, where he is diagnosed with tuberculosis.

1. What treatment regimen should be recommended for him?

2. If later it becomes clear that Mr. Green has multidrug-resistant tuberculosis, what other drug may be added?

3. How will you help Mr. Green understand the importance of taking his medications for 6 months?

# 15 Cold and Cough Agents

## CHAPTER OBJECTIVES

*After answering the following questions, the reader should be able to:*

1. Differentiate between the common cold and the flu
2. Differentiate between the specific types of cold and cough agents
3. Discuss the mode of action for each specific cold and cough agent

## KEY TERMS AND DEFINITIONS

*Complete the following by writing the answer in the space provided.*

1. Drugs that reduce the effects mediated by histamine, a chemical released by the body during allergic reactions, are

   called _____.

2. The _____ is a nonbacterial infection, characterized by a rapid onset of symptoms that include fever, headache, and fatigue.

3. Agents that increase the production and therefore presumably the clearance of mucus secretions in the respiratory

   tract, such as guaifenesin, are called _____ _____.

4. The best _____, especially with colds, is plain water and juices, avoiding caffeinated beverages, such as tea or colas, and beer or other alcoholic mixtures.

5. A nonbacterial respiratory tract infection, characterized by malaise and a runny nose, is called a(n)

   _____ _____.

6. Agents that facilitate removal of mucus by a lysing or mucolytic action, such as dornase alfa, are called

   _____ _____.

7. Drugs that suppress the cough reflex, and are useful in the presence of an irritating, persistent, nonproductive

   cough, are called _____.

8. Match the following signs and symptoms of the common cold and influenza:

   1. _____ Fever
   2. _____ No chills present
   3. _____ Headache
   4. _____ Nonproductive cough

   a. Cold
   b. Influenza

5. _____ Nasal congestion (common)

6. _____ Early and severe fatigue

7. _____ Sore throat (common)


The common cold is a nonbacterial upper respiratory tract infection (URI) that results in a general malaise and runny, stuffy nose. The many cold remedies available as over-the-counter (OTC) medications represent four classes of agents. These include sympathomimetics to decongest, antihistamines to dry secretions, expectorants to increase mucus clearance, and antitussives to suppress the cough reflex. Many preparations have two or more of these in combination. Each of these classes is discussed here briefly.

9. List four classes of drugs available to treat the common cold:

a. _____

b. _____

c. _____

d. _____

10. What are the indications for each of the four classes listed in question 9?

a. _____

b. _____

c. _____

d. _____

## SYMPATHOMIMETIC (ADRENERGIC) DECONGESTANTS

Sympathomimetics are used in cold remedies for their vasoconstriction ($\alpha$ receptor stimulation) or decongestant effect. Although most are given by topical application (nasal spray), some are systemic (oral) medications. Nasal sprays should be used only for a short time (1 to 2 days) because rebound nasal congestion can occur. Oral doses may provide better decongestion, but side effects of increased blood pressure and heart rate may occur.

11. Topical sympathomimetic _____ sprays or drops produce results faster than oral applications.

## ANTIHISTAMINE AGENTS

Histamine, released from mast cells and blood basophils, is a mediator of local inflammation. Its release can cause increased capillary permeability and dilation, itching, pain, and smooth muscle contraction. The inflammatory effects are produced when histamine stimulates cell surface histamine (H) receptors.

$H_1$ receptors are located in nerve endings, smooth muscle, and glandular cells. Stimulation of these receptors results in wheal-and-flare reactions in the skin. This is also called the *triple response,* causing redness, welt formation, and a reddish-white border. Bronchoconstriction, mucus secretion, and nasal congestion and irritation also occur with $H_1$ stimulation. Hypotension may occur in allergic anaphylaxis.

$H_2$ receptors regulate gastric acid secretion and a feedback mechanism for histamine release. They are located in the gastric region. HZ receptor antagonists block acid secretion in the stomach.

$H_3$ receptors, located in the airways, also may play a role in control of histamine synthesis and release.

Most "older" cold medications contain first-generation $H_1$ receptor antagonists. These agents block the bronchopulmonary and vascular actions of histamine and prevent rhinitis and urticaria (skin eruptions). They also have a sedative and anticholinergic effect. The sedative effect is thought to occur because of absorption into the brain. The anticholinergic effect contributes to upper airway drying. The airway drying may have a detrimental effect because secretion clearance is decreased. Duration of effect is usually 4 to 6 hours with first-generation drugs.

The second-generation $H_1$ receptor antagonists have less sedating and anticholinergic effects and last for 12 hours. They are more useful in the treatment of allergic rhinitis than colds. Both generations of drugs help control the allergic symptoms of sneezing and rhinorrhea. The various drugs available are listed in Table 15-3 in the textbook.

Ipratropium bromide nasal spray is an alternative to antihistamines for rhinorrhea. This anticholinergic agent is effective and shows no evidence of rebound congestion or systemic effects.

12. What are three effects of antihistamines?

    a. _____

    b. _____

    c. _____

13. The anticholinergic effect of first-generation $H_1$ receptor cold medications contributes to upper airway drying. Why is this a problem?

## EXPECTORANTS

Expectorants aid in the removal of secretions either by "breaking them up" (mucolytic) or by increasing mucus production (stimulant). There is controversy over the use of expectorants, as to who should use them and whether they are effective. Although some agents (guaifenesin) are considered safe and effective, little research has been done to demonstrate their effectiveness when used to treat the common cold. A list of some expectorants is given in Table 15-5 in the textbook.

14. What are three ways stimulant expectorants work?

    a. _____

    b. _____

    c. _____

15. The best expectorant for a simple cold is _____.

16. How do bland aerosols of saline increase sputum volume?

    a. _____

    b. _____

## COUGH SUPPRESSANTS (ANTITUSSIVES)

Coughing is a reflex defense mechanism used to clear the upper airway. Cough suppression may occur by depressing the cough center located in the medulla or by inhibiting the cough reflex at its source, the stretch receptors in the lungs.

Agents present in anticold compounds are listed in Box 15-1 in the textbook. Dextromethorphan and codeine are available in OTC preparations and are considered safe and effective. The following should be considered:

- Suppression of a dry hacking cough is appropriate and helpful.
- Suppression of a productive cough is not appropriate, especially when copious amounts of sputum is present.
- The combination of an expectorant and an antitussive probably doesn't make a lot of sense.

Table 15-6 in the textbook gives a list of cold remedies with the class of agents included in the compounds. Most are OTC compounds and need no prescription. The possibility of abuse with these remedies is real!

17. A common narcotic cough suppressant is _____.

18. True or False: Codeine does not produce analgesia in the adult.

19. True or False: It is appropriate to use a cough suppressant in diseases that have copious amounts of secretions such as cystic fibrosis to prevent irritation to the airway.

20. True or False: A cough suppressant is useful for a constant nonproductive cough that can lead to more coughing and lung irritation.

## COLD COMPOUNDS: TREATING A COLD

Every ingredient in cold remedies has potential problems, so remember to consider the undesirable effects posed by each ingredient.

And by the way, write them in the following blanks. *Complete the following by writing the undesirable effects of each category of ingredient in the space provided.*

21. Sympathomimetics

    a. _____

    b. _____

    c. _____

22. Antihistamines

    a. _____

    b. _____

    c. _____

23. Expectorants

    a. _____

24. Antitussives

    a. _____

Starve a cold, feed a fever. No, feed a cold, starve a fever. No, you can't cure a cold, so treat the symptoms and forget about the food!

## NATIONAL BOARD OF RESPIRATORY CARE–TYPE QUESTIONS

Don't forget fluids, rest, chicken soup, and the answers to NBRC-type questions.

1. Which of the following agents is useful in the presence of an irritating, persistent, nonproductive cough?
   a. Antitussive
   b. Expectorant
   c. Mucolytic expectorant
   d. Sympathomimetic

2. Which of the following symptoms is *not* associated with the flu?
   a. Fever
   b. Sore throat
   c. Fatigue
   d. Headache

3. An antihistamine used to treat a common cold is intended to:
   a. Decongest
   b. Suppress the cough reflex
   c. Dry secretions
   d. Increase mucus clearance

4. Which of the following is *not* true concerning the common cold?
   a. It is a nonbacterial respiratory tract infection.
   b. It is characterized by a runny nose.
   c. Nasal congestion is rare.
   d. Sneezing and sore throat are present.

5. An agent that increases the production and clearance of mucus secretions in the respiratory tract, such as guaifenesin, is called a:
   a. Antihistamine
   b. Antitussive
   c. Mucolytic expectorant
   d. Stimulant expectorant

6. Classes of drugs that are available to treat the common cold include:
   I. Sympathomimetics
   II. Antihistamines
   III. Expectorants
   IV. Antitussives
       a. I and II only
       b. II and III only
       c. I, III, and IV only
       d. I, II, III, and IV

7. A person has been diagnosed with a cold and also rhinitis. This would indicate that the patient has:
   a. Watery eyes
   b. Itchy throat
   c. Inflamed nasal passages
   d. Nonproductive cough

8. Nasal decongestion is achieved by sympathomimetics by stimulation of which receptor?
   a. $\beta_1$
   b. $\beta_2$
   c. $\alpha$
   d. $H_1$

9. The common cold is usually of _____ origin.
   a. Bacterial
   b. Viral
   c. Fungal
   d. Allergenic

10. Which of the following is *not* correct concerning oral administration of sympathomimetic decongestants?
    a. Slower onset of action
    b. Better decongestion
    c. Increased systemic side effects
    d. Increased incidence of rebound congestion

11. Which of the following classes of effects does *not* apply to antihistamines?
    a. Antihistaminic
    b. Sedative
    c. Anticholinergic
    d. Sympathomimetic

12. The anticholinergic effect of antihistamines on the upper airway results in:
    a. Bronchoconstriction
    b. Capillary leakage
    c. Drying
    d. Increased mucus production

13. Which of the following is recommended as being safe and effective as an expectorant?
    a. Terpin hydrate
    b. Guaifenesin
    c. Glycerol
    d. Iodine

14. The best expectorant for the cold is:
    a. Water
    b. Terpin hydrate
    c. Guaifenesin
    d. Glycerol

15. Which of the following side effects is most associated with an antihistamine?
    a. Tremor
    b. Drowsiness
    c. Hypertension
    d. Tachycardia

Your parents are away on a cruise and left you baby-sitting your little brother during spring break. Over the past few days he has developed a runny nose, is sneezing, and says he feels "icky." You take his temperature and it is 98.8° F.

1. What's your differential diagnosis?

2. What treatment would help him the most at present?

3. Being a good respiratory therapist, you anticipate that he may develop a cough that is dry and nonproductive, even though his temperature remains normal. You ask yourself, "Is there anything in his treatment regimen that can be changed so that I won't have to take him to the doctor?"

# 16 Selected Agents of Pulmonary Value

## CHAPTER OBJECTIVES

*After answering the following questions, the reader should be able to:*

1. Discuss the indication for $\alpha_1$-proteinase inhibitor
2. Recognize $\alpha_1$-proteinase inhibitor deficiency in a patient
3. List the $\alpha_1$-proteinase inhibitors that are available
4. List three types of formulations for nicotine replacement
5. Recognize the advantages and disadvantages of nicotine replacement
6. Discuss the indication for nitric oxide
7. Describe the effect of inhaled nitric oxide on a patient
8. List the two toxic products of nitric oxide
9. List the only inhaled antidiabetic agent available in the United States

## KEY TERMS AND DEFINITIONS

*Match the following definitions with their terms.*

1. _____ $\alpha_1$-Proteinase inhibitor (API) has altered electrophoretic properties and lower than normal serum concentrations

2. _____ Also known as $\alpha_1$-proteinase inhibitor, this inhibitor of trypsin may be deficient in patients with emphysema

3. _____ Undetectable API levels in the serum

4. _____ API is present in normal amounts, but does not function normally

5. _____ Individual has normal serum levels of API

a. $\alpha_1$-Antitrypsin
b. Deficient
c. Dysfunctional
d. Normal
e. Null

## $\alpha_1$-PROTEINASE INHIBITOR (HUMAN)

$\alpha_1$-proteinase inhibitor (API), also known as $\alpha_1$-antitrypsin ($\alpha_1$-AT) (Prolastin), is a drug prepared from the plasma of human donors. It is used to treat patients with a genetic defect resulting in decreased levels of $\alpha_1$-AT. Nonsmoking individuals with $\alpha_1$-AT levels below 35% develop panacinar emphysema between the ages of 30 and 50 years. Cigarette smokers develop greatly accelerated disease.

### $\alpha_1$-Antitrypsin Deficiency

$\alpha_1$-Antitrypsin deficiency is an autosomal recessive disorder that is estimated to account for 2% of all emphysema in the United States and is as common a genetic disorder among white individuals as cystic fibrosis. The development of emphysema at an early age, especially without cause (smoking, work history), should be suspect for $\alpha_1$-AT deficiency.

In the normal lung there's an enzyme called neutrophil elastase; its job is to cleave all forms of connective tissue and degrade elastic fiber. Neutrophil elastase is held in check by $\alpha_1$-antitrypsin. If there's a deficiency in $\alpha_1$-antitrypsin, the elastase "burns through" alveolar walls and the result is emphysema.

Prolastin therapy is indicated as long-term replacement therapy in patients who have a congenital $\alpha_1$-antitrypsin deficiency, with clinically demonstrated panacinar emphysema. By the time panacinar emphysema becomes evident the lungs have sustained structural damage. Prolastin won't reverse the damage, or improve lung function. Once the alveolar walls are gone, there's nothing that can be done about it.

## Indication for Drug Therapy

Prolastin ($\alpha_1$-proteinase inhibitor therapy) is indicated as chronic replacement therapy for individuals with severe $\alpha_1$-antitrypsin deficiency and panacinar emphysema. The drug cannot reverse lung damage, only help prevent further damage from occurring. Side effects from the weekly IV administration of Prolastin are minimal. The drug is very expensive, costing up to $40,000 per year.

6. $\alpha_1$-Antitrypsin deficiency, like cystic fibrosis, is an _____ _____ disorder.

7. True or False: The development of emphysema at an early age, especially with a smoking or work history, should be suspect for $\alpha_1$-antitrypsin deficiency.

8. An enzyme called neutrophil elastase, which can destroy alveolar walls, is held in check by

_____.

9. Explain the sequence of events leading to panacinar emphysema caused by $\alpha_1$-antitrypsin deficiency.

10. For individuals with congenital deficiency of API, with clinically demonstrable panacinar emphysema,

_____ is indicated as chronic replacement therapy.

## SMOKING CESSATION DRUG THERAPY

Nicotine stimulates the acetylcholine receptors at the autonomic ganglia of both the sympathetic and parasympathetic nervous systems. Nicotine stimulation results in discharge of both systems, with the sympathetic effects predominating. Release of epinephrine and norepinephrine from the adrenal medulla adds to these effects. Nicotine stimulates the cholinergic nicotine receptors in skeletal muscle, causing tremors and loss of hand steadiness. Nicotine also binds to receptors in the brain, resulting in respiratory stimulation, tremors, convulsions, nausea, and emesis. Central nervous system (CNS) binding also results in release of chemical mediators, such as dopamine, which give a feeling of pleasure, euphoria and well-being, enhanced concentration, cognitive arousal, and decrease of tension and anxiety.

Nicotine addiction is the basis for tobacco dependence. Sensitivity to nicotine in the CNS (nicotine addiction) is genetically determined. About 90% of smokers have the genetic substrate, resulting in some degree of nicotine addiction. Cessation of smoking is difficult for most individuals because of the development of nicotine withdrawal. Withdrawal involves physical symptoms including craving for nicotine, increased appetite, impaired concentration, nervousness, irritability, anxiety, and sleep disturbance.

Nicotine replacement therapy is initiated to replace the nicotine lost with smoking cessation. Over time, the gradual withdrawal of nicotine (decreased nicotine replacement) is better tolerated and withdrawal symptoms are not as bothersome. Forms of nicotine replacement include a transdermal patch, chewing gum, a nasal spray, an inhaler, and a lozenge.

11. What is the rationale for nicotine replacement therapy?

Nicotine polacrilex (Nicorette) gum releases nicotine that is absorbed through the membranes of the mouth. Use of nicotine nasal spray allows a rapid rise in plasma levels of nicotine. The nicotine inhaler delivers less nicotine than the other nicotine systems but simulates a cigarette and gives oral gratification. The nicotine transdermal patch can be applied to any clean, dry, hairless part of the body. Depending on the product, plasma levels will peak in 2 to 12 hours but remain elevated for a total of 24 hours. The nicotine lozenge (Commit) was approved by the U.S. Food and Drug Administration (FDA) in October 2002. It is an over-the-counter drug that can be used every 1–2 hours, with its use being tapered over a 12-week period. More than one form of nicotine replacement therapy can be used at one time to help maintain nicotine levels and to stimulate a nicotine "hit" similar to smoking a cigarette. An example would be the use of a transdermal patch with an inhaler as an adjunct therapy. Patients should not continue to smoke while using nicotine replacement therapy. Because nicotine is addictive, patients can become addicted to nicotine replacement therapy, just as they did to smoking cigarettes. Bupropion (Zyban) is an antidepressant and a nonnicotine agent used to aid smoking cessation. Varenicline (Chantix) inhibits the activation of $\alpha_4\beta_2$ receptors by nicotine, blocks the sensation produced by smoking, and breaks the cycle of nicotine additions. This works best by having the patient set a quit date for smoking. Starting Chantix 1 week before the quit date is best. This is a 12-week-long treatment process.

12. Why might the nicotine inhaler be preferred to gum and nasal spray?

13. True or False: Patients should not continue to smoke while using nicotine replacement therapy.

14. True or False: In general, if a person has not made significant progress toward abstinence from smoking by week 7, Zyban should be discontinued.

15. Chantix is used to block receptors for _____, reducing the sensation produced by smoking.

## NITRIC OXIDE

Nitric oxide (NO) is a product of endothelial cells. Originally called endothelium-derived relaxing factor, nitric oxide is a vasodilator. Inhaled nitric oxide (INO) is a gas that can be used to cause pulmonary vasodilation. Because of the rapid deactivation of NO, as a result of binding to hemoglobin, NO is a selective pulmonary vasodilator. NO is approved for use in neonates with hypoxic respiratory failure to reduce pulmonary hypertension. The recommended dosage of NO is 20 parts per million (ppm). Increased concentrations increase the risk of lung injury by NO, the likelihood of elevated nitrogen dioxide ($NO_2$) levels, and the development of methemoglobinemia. $NO_2$ is a strong oxidizer, causing cellular lipid peroxidation. Methemoglobin results when iron in the hemoglobin molecule is changed from the normal ferrous (2+) state to the ferric (3+) state by the attachment of NO. Methemoglobin cannot carry oxygen and shifts the oxygen dissociation curve to the left, thus limiting oxygen availability to the tissues. INO is approved for neonates (>34 weeks of gestation) with hypoxic respiratory failure associated with evidence of pulmonary hypertension.

16. Nitric oxide is a gas that can be inhaled to cause _____ vasodilation.

17. Because of the rapid deactivation of nitric oxide, the result of its binding to hemoglobin, nitric oxide is a

_____ pulmonary vasodilator.

18. Indications for INO is for neonates with a gestational age of _____ weeks.

19. The recommended dosage of INO is _____ parts per million.

20. Administration of INO above the recommended dose can cause increased levels of _____

_____ and _____.

21. According to the American Academy of Pediatrics, sample gas for analysis should be drawn

_____ the wye adaptor, proximal to the patient.

22. True or False: Blood methemoglobin levels should be drawn every other day.

23. True or False: Weaning from nitric oxide should be gradual to prevent arterial desaturation and pulmonary hypertension.

24. True or False: The dose of nitric oxide should always start at 40 ppm and can be increased to 80 ppm if no clinical signs of pulmonary vasodilation occur.

25. True or False: Because INO has a short half-life, as soon as the INO is discontinued, pulmonary vasodilation ends.

26. True or False: Some systemic vasodilation occurs at higher doses, leading to hypotension

27. True or False: The higher the fraction of inspired oxygen ($Fi_{O2}$) the greater the amount of oxidation of nitric oxide to nitrogen dioxide.

28. INO becomes inactive when it enters the red blood cell and attaches to _____.

29. Some endogenous nitric oxide is exhaled from the lungs after being converted to _____ within the red blood cells.

30. Improvement of arterial oxygen pressure ($Pa_{O2}$) with INO is due to _____ of pulmonary

blood vessels and improved _____ – _____ matching.

## INSULIN HUMAN (rDNA ORIGIN)

Insulin human (rDNA origin) (Exubera) is an orally inhaled insulin medication. Not a respiratory drug but side effects such as bronchospasm and reduction in lung function is possible. The drug is used for type 1 and 2 diabetes for adults 18 years of age and older. It comes in powdered form and should be taken immediately before meals. Patients with uncontrolled lung disease should not take Exubera because of effects on lung function and diffusing capacity. It is also contraindicated in smokers or patients who have quit smoking less than 6 months before starting therapy. Patients taking bronchodilators should take the prescribed dose 30 minutes before Exubera.

31. A possible respiratory side effect of Exubera is _____ and reduction in lung function.

32. Exubera is contraindicated for:

    a. _____

    b. _____

33. When should a diabetic patient take Exubera?

## NATIONAL BOARD OF RESPIRATORY CARE–TYPE QUESTIONS

1. What type of disorder is $\alpha_1$-antitrypsin deficiency? (*Hint:* Think of cystic fibrosis.)
   a. Autosomal recessive
   b. Disomonal
   c. Trisomy 13
   d. XY recessive

2. Which statement is *true* regarding $\alpha_1$-antitrypsin ($\alpha_1$-AT) deficiency?
   a. It is generally seen at a later age, as a result of smoking.
   b. It is caused by excessive exposure to asbestos at an early age.
   c. It develops at an early age among people without cause (smoking, relevant work history).
   d. It develops in patients >65 years of age with a history of exposure to wood dust.

3. What drug is indicated as a chronic replacement therapy for individuals with congenital deficiency or $\alpha_1$-proteinase deficiency and who have panacinar emphysema?
   a. Proteinastin
   b. Prolastin
   c. Antitrypsinogen
   d. Nicotrypsin

4. What is the purpose of nicotine replacement therapy?
   a. To reduce the number of cigarettes smoked by a patient
   b. To reduce the food cravings of a smoking patient who is cutting down on the number of cigarettes smoked per day
   c. To replace the nicotine lost with smoking cessation
   d. To help eliminate nicotine from the body during weaning from cigarette smoking

5. Which of the following methods of administering nicotine would simulate a cigarette and give oral gratification?
   a. Nicotine gum
   b. Nicotine nasal spray
   c. Nicotine patch
   d. Nicotine inhaler

6. Bupropion (Zyban) contains which of the following?
   I. Nonnicotine agent to help reduce smoking
   II. Antidepressant
   III. Analgesic
   IV. Nicotine
      a. I and II only
      b. II and III only
      c. I and III only
      d. I, II, and III only

7. Before prescribing Varenicline (Chantix) to a patient who is currently smoking, you should have the patient set a

   quit date and start the medication _____ week(s) before this date.
   a. 1
   b. 2
   c. 3
   d. 4

8. The indication for INO is for neonates with a gestational age of:
   a. >34 weeks
   b. <24 weeks
   c. <27 weeks
   d. <31 weeks

9. INO is considered to be a selective pulmonary artery vasodilator because:
   a. It is inhaled.
   b. The nitric oxide rapidly deactivates once it attaches to hemoglobin.
   c. A large dose is administered and the oxygen concentration is high.
   d. It converts to nitrogen dioxide, which remains in the lung.

10. The recommended dose of INO is:
   a. 80 ppm
   b. 60 ppm
   c. 40 ppm
   d. 20 ppm

11. Administration of NO above the recommended levels can increase levels of:
    I. Methemoglobin
    II. Nitrogen dioxide
    III. Sulfhemoglobin
    IV. Nitrohemoglobin
        a. I and II only
        b. II and III only
        c. I, III, and IV only
        d. II and IV only

12. About _____% of smokers have the genetic substrate resulting in some degree of nicotine addiction.
    a. 10%
    b. 40%
    c. 60%
    d. 90%

13. Even though Exubera is not a respiratory drug, side effects that are possible from inhalation of the drug include:
    a. Bronchospasm
    b. Excessive secretions in lower airway
    c. Reduced secretions in upper airway
    d. Pulmonary artery vasoconstriction

14. Contraindication to Exubera includes which of the following?
    a. Diabetes type 2
    b. Diabetes type 1
    c. Smokers
    d. Congestive heart failure (CHF)

15. According to the American Academy of Pediatrics, sampling of gas containing NO for analysis of a patient on mechanical ventilation should take place:
    a. On the inspiratory side of the patient circuit, where INO first enters the circuit
    b. On the expiratory side of the patient circuit
    c. Before the wye adaptor, proximal to the patient
    d. On the expiratory side of the patient circuit, just before the exhalation valve of the ventilator

You are conducting a smoking cessation class at a local lung association. One of the participants is the president of a local university. She works an average of 60 hr/week and is widely known, indicating a high level of stress. She uses smoking as a means to reduce stress but wants to quit.

1. She asks you to recommend the method that would best suit her lifestyle. What would you recommend?

2. After some use of the transdermal patch she complains that she has skin irritation where she places the patch each day. What would you recommend?

3. Your patient is a heavy smoker (about 40 cigarettes a day). Would you give her any other advice and/or instructions?

4. After 2 weeks on the transdermal patch she complains of feeling depressed and feels she cannot continue with the smoking cessation program. What would you suggest?

# 17 Neonatal and Pediatric Aerosolized Drug Therapy

## CHAPTER OBJECTIVES

*After answering the following questions, the reader should be able to:*

1. Explain off-label use of aerosolized medications
2. Describe the advantages and disadvantages of aerosol delivery
3. List and describe the most important factors affecting neonatal and pediatric aerosol drug delivery
4. Describe the clinical response of neonatal and pediatric patients to aerosolized drugs
5. Describe special situations related to selection of delivery devices for neonatal and pediatric patients
6. Explain lung deposition of inhaled drugs in pediatric and neonatal intubated patients

## KEY TERMS AND DEFINITIONS

*Match the following definitions with their terms.*

1. _____ A child between the ages of 1 month and 1 year

2. _____ Drugs are dosed until a certain blood level is reached; therefore therapeutic effects and side effects are related to the drug concentration in the blood

3. _____ The dose actually reaching the trachea and beyond

4. _____ The period of time between birth and the first month of life

5. _____ Refers to the period of time between 1 month and 18 years of age

6. _____ The dose released by the aerosol device

7. _____ The dose reaching the patient's mouth or artificial airway

8. _____ Drugs are dosed until the desired effect is achieved or unacceptable side effects or toxicity occur

9. _____ The dose in the delivery device

10. _____ Use of drugs with no U.S. Food and Drug Administration (FDA)-approved labeling

a. Emitted dose
b. Infant
c. Inhaled or delivered dose
d. Lung dose
e. Neonatal
f. Nominal dose
g. Off-label
h. Pediatric
i. Target concentration
j. Target effect

## OFF-LABEL USE OF DRUGS IN NEONATAL AND PEDIATRIC PATIENTS

Many aerosolized drugs, when receiving FDA approval, are not approved for use with infants and children. The use of drugs not officially approved for specific ages or conditions is called "off-label" use. Once a drug is approved by the FDA, it may be prescribed by a licensed physician as he or she sees fit. The FDA cannot regulate how a drug is used medically; and therefore off-label use is not illegal. However, some general guidelines should be followed. The therapy should be considered reasonable and safe, parameters used for monitoring during therapy should be predetermined, and the drug should be prescribed according to standards of care. In general, drug dosing is based on one of two strategies. Dosing until a desired blood level is achieved is referred to as *target concentration dosing*. Dosing until the desired effect results is called *target effect dosing*. The latter dosing strategy is normally used for aerosol therapy.

11. List three general guidelines for off-label drug use:

   a. _____

   b. _____

   c. _____

## ADVANTAGES OF AEROSOL DELIVERY IN NEONATAL AND PEDIATRIC PATIENTS

Compared to systemic drug administration, aerosol drug delivery offers the same general advantages for neonatal and pediatric patients as it does for adults.
- Feasible route of administration
- Rapid response
- Painless, safe, and decreased complications
- Potential for smaller doses
- Direct organ targeting with reduced systemic exposure

12. What is the major advantage of using inhaled aerosols in neonatal and pediatric patients?

*Fill in the following table, indicating the differences between neonatal and adult anatomy and respiratory parameters that would affect aerosol penetration and deposition.*

|                          | Neonate | Adult |
|--------------------------|---------|-------|
| 13. Tracheal length      |         |       |
| 14. Tidal volume         |         |       |
| 15. Minute ventilation   |         |       |
| 16. Respiratory rate     |         |       |
| 17. Inspiratory flow rate|         |       |

## FACTORS AFFECTING NEONATAL AND PEDIATRIC AEROSOL DRUG DELIVERY

Although the same mechanisms of aerosol penetration and deposition apply to both pediatric and adult populations, functional and structural features of the immature airway (in patients less than 9 years of age) also may have an effect on aerosol deposition. Smaller airway diameters throughout the pulmonary system may be a major factor resulting in decreased aerosol deposition in the lower airways. Decreased inspiratory flow rate, smaller tidal volumes, and breathing pattern contribute to decreased lung levels of inhaled drugs, especially in infants and neonates. Delivery devices, in particular reservoir devices, also can have an effect on the amount of drug available to the lungs. In adults, use of reservoirs tends to increase the amount of drug delivery; in small children, this use tends to decrease the amount of delivered drug.

The following four terms help clarify what is meant by specific drug dosages:

- The *nominal dose* is the amount of drug in the delivery device. In the small volume nebulizer (SVN), it is the amount of drug placed in the nebulizer. For the metered dose inhaler (MDI), it is the amount of drug in the metering valve; for the dry powder inhaler (DPI), it is the amount in the blister pack.
- The *emitted dose* is the amount of drug produced by the delivery device. The emitted dose is significantly lower than the nominal dose for the SVN because of "dead volume" in the nebulizer. It is similar to the nominal dose for the MDI and DPI.
- The *delivered dose* or *inhaled dose* is the amount of drug reaching the airway (mouth, nose, endotracheal tube). This dose is significantly less than the emitted dose for the SVN because it is an open system and drug is lost to the atmosphere. The delivered dose is significantly less than the emitted dose for an MDI with a holding chamber. It is similar to the emitted dose for the MDI and DPI placed directly in the mouth.
- The *lung dose* is the actual amount of drug that reaches the trachea and subsequent airways. It is less than the delivered dose for the SVN, MDI, and DPI because some (a great deal) is always lost in the mouth. It is important to use correct terms when discussing aerosolized drug delivery. The typical lung dose in adults is 10 to 15% of the nominal dose, whereas in children it may be only 6%. Age (weight) adjustments for the amount of drug given are common for parenterally administered medications. It may not be applicable for inhaled medications. Research indicates that lung dose of aerosolized medications is self-limiting in the immature airway, and deposition is proportionally less than in adults.

18. List three causes of decreased aerosolized drug deposition in the neonatal and pediatric lung:

    a. _____

    b. _____

    c. _____

19. True or False: The nominal dose is the amount of drug in the nebulizer (SVN) or in the metering valve (MDI); for a DPI it is the amount of drug in the blister pack.

20. True or False: The emitted dose is greater than the nominal dose.

**Effect of Age on the Aerosol Lung Dose**

21. The actual dose of an inhaled aerosol drug in neonates and infants can be as low as less than

    _____ in neonates and approximately _____ in the young child, compared with the traditional 10% to 15% cited for adults.

22. Lower _____ in the lung helps prevent smaller patients from receiving high drug per kilogram of body weight.

**Effect of Small Tidal Volumes, Short Respiratory Cycles, and Low Flow Rates**

23. List three reasons why children inhale a smaller percentage of the emitted dose from either a small volume nebulizer or MDI with a reservoir device.

    a. _____

    b. _____

    c. _____

24. What is the ideal volume for a spacer device for an infant?

*The following is a list of factors that may affect the dose inhaled from a reservoir chamber by neonatal and pediatric patients. Identify each as either (a) a mechanical and design factor or (b) a patient factor.*

25. _____ Electrostatic charge on plastic devices

26. _____ Tidal volume

27. _____ Presence of inspiratory valve

28. _____ Inspiratory flow rate

29. _____ Amount of dead volume in mouthpiece

a. Mechanical and design factor
b. Patient factor

## CLINICAL RESPONSE TO AEROSOLIZED DRUGS IN NEONATAL AND PEDIATRIC PATIENTS

Although the percentage of drug delivery has been shown to be self-limiting in young children, actual required drug dose should be evaluated by clinical response. Adult and neonatal tissues do not always have the same response and may require adjusted drug dosing. Studies from the 1970s seemed to indicate that infants younger than 18 months did not respond to adrenergic bronchodilators. The authors speculated that there was either poor smooth muscle development or bronchial obstruction due to secretions and airway edema. However, studies from the 1990s have shown dose-related improvements in respiratory mechanics with administration of aerosolized bronchodilators. More research must be conducted to determine appropriate drug doses in young children, infants, and neonates.

30. Why might a younger patient (<18 months of age) not have as great of a clinical response to medication as compared with an older child?

## CHOICE OF DELIVERY DEVICE IN NEONATAL AND PEDIATRIC PATIENTS

Current guidelines present the following recommendations for the use of SVNs, MDIs, and DPIs in neonatal and pediatric patients. SVNs can be used in any age group. Care must be taken with inline ventilator use. Masks are required for those unable to use a mouthpiece. An MDI with endotracheal tube (ETT) also can be used with any age group. An MDI with a mask should be used in patients up to age 4 years. After age 4 years, an MDI with a reservoir and mouthpiece can be used. MDIs without a reservoir, breath-activated MDIs, and DPIs should not be used in children younger than 5 years. These are guidelines; appropriate clinical judgment must be used to determine the most appropriate method of administration.

*List the type of aerosol system that can be used for each of the age groups listed:*

31. Neonate: _____

32. Child ≥ 5 years of age: _____

**168**

33. Child ≥ 4 years of age: _____

34. Child ≤ 4 years of age: _____

35. Administration of nebulized aerosol using the "blow-by" technique can reduce the inhaled drug mass in a

    pediatric patient as much as _____.

36. Why can't a DPI be used by children younger than 5 years?

## AEROSOL ADMINISTRATION IN INTUBATED NEONATAL AND PEDIATRIC PATIENTS

37. List three potential problems that may occur with an externally powered nebulizer placed in-line on a pediatric and
    neonatal ventilator:

    a. _____

    b. _____

    c. _____

38. Aerosol delivery may be less effective with _____ ventilation versus mechanical ventilation.

Remember: SVNs are typically used with a facemask that the caregiver, parent, or child can hold. Crying reduces tidal volume and lung deposition; it can help to make a game of it (e.g., the child pretends to be an astronaut, pilot, etc.).

## NATIONAL BOARD OF RESPIRATORY CARE–TYPE QUESTIONS

1. A person in the first 4 weeks of postnatal life is correctly termed which of the following?
   a. Postmature neonate
   b. Neonate
   c. Infant
   d. Baby

2. Which of the following is the route of administration of choice for delivering medication to the lungs of a child?
   a. IV
   b. Topical
   c. Oral
   d. Aerosol

3. Which aerosol delivery device(s) can be used to treat a neonate?
   a. SVN
   b. MDI through endotracheal tube
   c. MDI with spacer
   d. Both a and b

4. Which aerosol delivery devices can be used to treat a 5-year-old patient?
   a. SVN
   b. MDI with spacer
   c. DPI
   d. All the above

5. Aerosol deposition in the neonate may be affected by which of the following?
    I. Decreased inspiratory flow rate
    II. Smaller tidal volume
    III. Smaller airways
    IV. Shorter respiratory cycle
        a. I and II only
        b. II and III only
        c. I, II, and IV only
        d. I, II, III, and IV

6. Which of the following applies to a DPI?
    a. Requires that the user generate >60 L/min of flow
    b. Should be used only with a spacer
    c. Can be done with an endotracheal tube
    d. All of the above

7. The dose of drug that is released from the aerosol device is called the:
    a. Inhaled dose
    b. Target dose
    c. Emitted dose
    d. Lung dose

8. Which of the following is *not* a general guideline for off-label drug use?
    a. The therapy should be reasonable and safe.
    b. Parameters used for monitoring during therapy should be predetermined.
    c. The drug is prescribed according to the standards of care.
    d. The drug can be used only for 2 days of therapy.

9. What is the major advantage of administering inhaled aerosols to neonatal and pediatric patients?
    a. It delivers a greater dose compared with systemic administration of drugs.
    b. It avoids systemic factors that can affect oral or injectable drug therapy.
    c. It prolongs the half-life of the drug, which therefore remains in the body longer.
    d. It produces fewer toxic effects in other organs, and the therapeutic index is greater.

10. You are administering a small volume nebulizer aerosol to a 9-year-old asthmatic. The amount of albuterol you place in the SVN is called the:
    a. Nominal dose
    b. Lung dose
    c. Effective dose
    d. Target dose

11. The delivered dose of medication from an SVN, MDI, or DPI is greater than the _____ dose.
    a. Emitted
    b. Lung
    c. Target
    d. Specific

12. The actual dose of an inhaled aerosol drug in neonates can be as low as:
    a. 5%
    b. 10%
    c. <1%
    d. 15%

13. Which of the following patient factors does *not* affect the dose inhaled from a reservoir chamber?
    a. Inspiratory flow rate
    b. Tidal volume
    c. Respiratory cycle
    d. Position of the patient in bed

14. Administration of nebulized aerosol with a facemask using the "blow-by" technique can reduce the inhaled drug mass in a pediatric patient as much as:
    a. 50%
    b. 10%
    c. 5%
    d. 1%

15. A 6-month-old with bronchiolitis has been ordered to receive an albuterol aerosol treatment. Which of the following would be the best aerosol delivery system to use?
    a. MDI with reservoir
    b. SVN with mouthpiece
    c. MDI or DPI with reservoir
    d. SVN with mask

16. When using an externally powered nebulizer in-line on a mechanical ventilator, which of the following are potential problems that can occur?
    I. Increased volume or pressure
    II. Bias flow interference with patient triggering
    III. Increase levels of positive end-expiratory pressure (PEEP)
    IV. Variable fraction of inspired oxygen ($FI_{O2}$)
        a. I and II only
        b. II and III only
        c. I, II, and IV only
        d. I, II, III, and IV

An 18-month-old child in intensive care unit has been admitted with a history of fever, cough, wheezing, and congestion over the last 3 days. She has been ordered to receive albuterol via aerosol therapy.

1. What delivery devices are available to you?

2. The child is not intubated. Which method of delivery would you select? Justify your selection.

3. As you begin the treatment she begins to cry and thrashes around on your lap. What should you do?

4. The child has deteriorated over the past 12 hours and is electively intubated and placed on mechanical ventilation. Albuterol treatments are continued on a regimen of every 2 to 4 hours. Which delivery device would you consider using?

# 18 Skeletal Muscle Relaxants (Neuromuscular Blocking Agents)

## CHAPTER OBJECTIVES

*After answering the following questions, the reader should be able to:*

1. Define neuromuscular blocking agents (NMBAs) and their mechanism of action
2. List the classes of NMBA available and describe the differences amongst the agents
3. Explain the neuromuscular physiology of nerve conduction
4. Describe the pharmacology of NMBAs
5. Identify potential drug interactions and complications of NMBAs
6. Review indications for NMBAs and monitoring parameters

## KEY TERMS AND DEFINITIONS

*Match the following definitions with their terms.*

1. _____ This is the accidental inhalation of food particles, fluids, or gastric contents into the lungs

2. _____ One of the basic functional units of the nervous system that is specialized to transmit electrical nerve impulses and carry information from one part of the body to another; it consists of a cell body, axons, and dendrites

3. _____ A pneumonia that is acquired in a healthcare setting

4. _____ A chemical that is released from a nerve ending to transmit an impulse from a nerve cell to another nerve, muscle, organ, or other tissue

5. _____ This substance or drug has the ability to cause total or partial loss of memory

6. _____ Involuntary contractions or twitching of groups of muscle fibers

7. _____ An enzyme that breaks down the neurotransmitter acetylcholine at the synaptic cleft, so that the next nerve impulse can be transmitted across the synaptic gap

8. _____ The production of a restful state of mind, particularly by the use of drugs that have a calming effect, relieving anxiety and tension

9. _____ An autoimmune neuromuscular disorder characterized by chronic fatigue and exhaustion of muscles

a. Acetylcholinesterase
b. Amnestic properties
c. Aspiration
d. Fasciculations
e. Myasthenia gravis
f. Neuromuscular blocking agent (NMBA)
g. Neuron (nerve cell)
h. Neurotransmitter
i. Nosocomial pneumonia
j. Sedation
k. Status asthmaticus
l. Status epilepticus

10. _____ A person having at least 30 minutes of continuous seizure activity without full recovery between seizures

11. _____ A substance that interferes with the neural transmission between motor neurons and skeletal muscles

12. _____ An attack of asthma lasting for more than 24 hours

## USES OF NEUROMUSCULAR BLOCKING AGENTS

Neuromuscular blocking agents are drugs used to cause skeletal muscle paralysis. The nondepolarizing blockers work by competitive inhibition for acetylcholine receptors at the neuromuscular junction. The depolarizing blocker succinylcholine exerts its effect by occupying the acetylcholine receptors, depolarizing the postjunctional membrane, and preventing repolarization from occurring. The neuromuscular blocking agents are used primarily to do the following:
- To facilitate endotracheal intubation
- For muscle relaxation during surgery, particularly of the thorax and abdomen
- To enhance patient–ventilator synchrony
- To reduce intracranial pressure in intubated patients with uncontrolled intracranial pressure
- To reduce oxygen consumption
- To terminate convulsive status epilepticus and tetanus in patients refractory to other therapies
- To facilitate procedures or diagnostic studies
- For selected patients who must remain immobile (e.g., trauma patients)

13. Describe the difference between a depolarizing and nondepolarizing agent.

14. Name the only depolarizing drug currently available.

## PHYSIOLOGY OF THE NEUROMUSCULAR JUNCTION

For a quick review of the peripheral nervous system (PNS) see Figure 18-1. The PNS is subdivided into the autonomic nervous system and the somatic nervous system. The somatic or skeletal muscle nervous system innervates striated muscle, including the diaphragm. Nerve stimulation results in release of acetylcholine at the neuromuscular junction, muscle depolarization, and contraction. During repolarization the muscle relaxes and is again ready for the next stimulus. The somatic nervous system is under voluntary control. The autonomic nervous system has two branches: the parasympathetic and the sympathetic nervous systems. These nerves innervate smooth muscles that are under involuntary (automatic) control. Both the parasympathetic and the sympathetic systems release acetylcholine at the neuroganglia, whereas only the parasympathetic system releases acetylcholine at the neuroeffector site. The sympathetic nervous system releases norepinephrine. Although neuromuscular blocking agents act on the acetylcholine receptors at the neuromuscular junction, they also affect other acetylcholine receptors. This is the reason for some of the side effects seen with the use of these agents.

15. Circle the correct answer: The somatic motor nervous system, or skeletal muscle system, controls (involuntary/voluntary) movement whereas the autonomic nervous system controls (involuntary/voluntary) movement.

16. The transmission of nerve conduction in skeletal muscle is chemically mediated by the neurotransmitter

    _____.

17. Acetylcholine is then broken down and inactivated by the enzyme _____ allowing the muscle fiber to repolarize.

18. There are two phases to muscle stimulation: _____ is the phase in which contraction of

    the muscle occurs. _____ is the phase during which the muscle fiber can be restimulated. Until this phase occurs the muscle is refractory.

Therefore muscle contraction can be blocked, causing paralysis, by the following:

- Competitive inhibition: the binding and blocking of the acetylcholine receptors without depolarization; this is the action of the nondepolarizing agents.
- Prolonged occupation and persistent binding of the acetylcholine receptors, resulting in sustained depolarization of the neuromuscular junction; this is the action of the depolarizing agents.

## NONDEPOLARIZING AGENTS

Nondepolarizing agents are so named because stimulation and depolarization of the muscle never occur. The nondepolarizing agents work by competitive inhibition of acetylcholine at the neuromuscular receptor sites. Although the various blockers may work by different methods, they all prevent the process of muscle depolarization; thus their name, nondepolarizers. Their effect is dose related, with increased doses resulting in increased effect. The drugs should be given by IV administration. Tubocurarine (curare) exemplifies the nondepolarizing blocking agents. IV administration causes effects in 1 to 2 minutes, with maximal effects in 2 to 10 minutes. Initial effects include drooping of the eyelids and inability to lift the head. This is followed by paralysis of the legs and arms. And finally there is loss of diaphragmatic function indicated by a lack of movement of the abdomen as the diaphragm moves. Maximal paralysis lasts for 35 minutes. Recovery begins in the reverse order of muscle paralysis and may take several hours. Factors such as increased age and hepatic and renal failure prolong the duration of the agents.

Because the nondepolarizing blocking agents are not site specific to the neuromuscular junction but instead compete with other acetylcholine receptors, there are some side effects that may occur. These include tachycardia and increased blood pressure. All nondepolarizing blocking agents cause histamine release from mast cells, which may lead to bronchoconstriction and hypotension. Another hazard of using nondepolarizing agents is inadequate ventilation. Muscle paralysis leads to apnea. Adequate ventilation must be supplied until adequate spontaneous ventilation can resume.

Muscle paralysis caused by nondepolarizing blocking agents can be reversed with the use of anticholinesterases such as neostigmine, edrophonium and pyridostigmine. Cholinesterase inactivates acetylcholine. If cholinesterase is blocked, acetylcholine is able to increase at the neuromuscular junction and compete with the nondepolarizing agent. This results in acetylcholine overriding the effects of the neuromuscular blocking agent, causing depolarization and muscle contraction. The reversing agents also increase the effects of acetylcholine at parasympathetic ganglia and produce cholinergic side effects including bradycardia and increased salivation. Use of a vagolytic agent (atropine) helps to decrease these side effects.

19. What is the first indication that paralysis is taking effect when administering a nondepolarizing agent?

20. What would be the first indication that the nondepolarizing agent is reversing or wearing off?

21. What are two concerns to respiratory therapists when administering nondepolarizing agents?

22. What type of drug would reverse nondepolarizing agents?

23. Which reversal agent is used to treat myasthenia gravis?

24. List two side effects of nondepolarizing agents:

   a. _____

   b. _____

25. Which neuromuscular blocking agent would not be recommended for a patient with asthma?

26. What neuromuscular blocking agent would not be recommended for a patient with high blood pressure and tachycardia?

## DEPOLARIZING AGENTS

Succinylcholine is the only depolarizing agent available in the United States. Its use results in total paralysis in 60 to 90 seconds and lasts for 10 to 15 minutes, making it ideal for intubation. Its mechanism of action causes refractory depolarization of the postsynaptic muscle membrane at the neuromuscular junction. The depolarization state continues until the drug is removed. The drug causes an initial muscle contraction followed by flaccid paralysis. Use of the drug causes stimulation of the autonomic nervous system, resulting in tachycardia and increased blood pressure in adults and bradycardia and decreased blood pressure in babies. Repeat doses may cause bradycardia and hypotension in adults also. As with nondepolarizing agents, succinylcholine causes the release of histamine. There is no effective reversing agent for succinylcholine, except to wait for it to leave the receptor site.

Adverse effects with the use of succinylcholine include muscle pain and soreness, transient serum potassium elevation, increased intraocular pressure, and increased intracranial pressure in patients with cerebral edema or head trauma. A condition known as malignant hyperthermia can develop in genetically susceptible individuals. This condition results in hyperthermia, acidosis, cardiovascular collapse, and death if not corrected. Muscle necrosis can occur in patients with myopathies or muscular dystrophies.

Much of the dose of succinylcholine (95% to 98%) is inactivated before it reaches the neuromuscular junction. Deactivation is accomplished by a plasma cholinesterase known as pseudocholinesterase. Individuals with a genetic variation causing them to have little or no pseudocholinesterase will require hours of ventilator support until the drug leaves the receptor, is redistributed, and is metabolized or excreted. Laboratory tests are available to check for these atypical cases.

27. The main indication for use of succinylcholine is _____.

28. Depolarization is initially indicated by _____ followed by flaccid paralysis.

29. List three side effects of succinylcholine that occur in most adult patients:

    a. _____

    b. _____

    c. _____

## NEUROMUSCULAR BLOCKING AGENTS AND MECHANICAL VENTILATION

The use of nondepolarizing blocking agents is appropriate in mechanically ventilated patients who are breathing out of synchrony (fighting) with the ventilator. Their use will help to increase ventilation and oxygenation and decrease peak ventilation pressure and work of breathing. Paralyzed patients must be closely monitored because there is absence of spontaneous ventilation. Use may be indicated for patients with the following conditions:
- Status asthmaticus
- Ventilator modes with prolonged inspiratory time (pressure-controlled inverse ratio ventilation)
- Status epilepticus
- Tetanus
- Neuromuscular toxins (strychnine poisoning)

It must be noted that use of the neuromuscular blocking agents only causes muscle paralysis; they do not provide sedation (remove conscious awareness) or pain relief (analgesia). Use of neuromuscular blockers without proper sedation and pain control is unacceptable. Prolonged use of neuromuscular blocking agents can lead to muscle atrophy (decrease in size) and myopathy (an abnormal condition of muscle weakness and wasting with histological changes within the muscle mass). It may take months to recover from these conditions.

Some disease states and drugs influence the action of neuromuscular blocking agents. In some situations they act synergistically with each other, whereas in others they are antagonistic. The aminoglycoside antibiotics and immunosuppressants potentiate the neuromuscular blockade. Theophylline antagonizes neuromuscular blockade. Alkalosis and hypercalcemia are known to inhibit the effects of blockade.

30. Retention of secretions is thought to increase the incidence of _____

_____ in patients receiving neuromuscular blockade for a prolonged period.

31. In paralyzed patients receiving mechanical ventilation, elevating the head can reduce the risk of

_____.

32. Remember that neuromuscular blocking agents only cause muscle paralysis. What should be administered to remove conscious awareness and/or pain relief?

33. For intubation, a short-acting neuromuscular blocking agent and a sedative that has _____ properties should be administered.

## MONITORING OF NEUROMUSCULAR BLOCKADE

With brief periods of paralysis, neuromuscular function can be assessed by voluntary actions such as spontaneous respiratory rate, maximal inspiratory force, vital capacity, hand grip, and the patient's ability to hold the head off the bed for 5 seconds. A more precise method to assess function is achieved through peripheral nerve stimulation.

34. True or False: Direct observation of muscle activity provides the simplest means of monitoring adequacy of blockade.

35. List, in order of occurrence, the sequence of paralysis of the skeletal muscles that can be monitored physically.

36. During brief periods of paralysis two simple measures of voluntary muscular functions include subjective assessments such as:

a. _____

b. _____

37. True or False: When using the train of four monitoring technique, the fewer twitches that occur when a stimulus is applied the greater the degree of neuromuscular blockade.

## NATIONAL BOARD OF RESPIRATORY CARE–TYPE QUESTIONS

1. Which of the following is *not* an indication for a neuromuscular blocking agent?
   a. Endotracheal extubation
   b. Muscle paralysis during surgery
   c. To facilitate mechanical ventilation
   d. Endotracheal intubation

2. If a mechanically ventilated patient is receiving vecuronium, the patient should also receive which of the following?
   I. Sedation
   II. Analgesics
   III. Frequent suctioning
   IV. Bronchodilator therapy

a. I and II only
b. I and III only
c. II, III, and IV only
d. I, II, III, and IV

3. Muscle contraction occurs during which of the following?
a. Apolarization
b. Depolarization
c. Repolarization
d. Myelination

4. The only depolarizing drug is which of the following?
a. Tubocurarine
b. Doxacurium
c. Pancuronium
d. Succinylcholine

5. Muscle paralysis caused by nondepolarizing blocking agents can be reversed by which of the following?
a. Cholinesterase
b. Cholinesterase inhibitors
c. Parasympatholytics
d. Sympathomimetics

6. The transmission of nerve conduction in skeletal muscle is chemically mediated by which of the following neurotransmitters?
a. Acetylcholine (ACh)
b. Pseudocholinesterase
c. Anticholinesterase
d. Norepinephrine

7. Which of the following drugs can reverse the effects of pancuronium?
a. Decamethonium
b. Neostigmine
c. Prostigmine
d. Reversostigmine

8. An asthmatic patient is about to be intubated and placed on mechanical ventilation. Which of the following neuromuscular blocking agents should *not* be administered?
a. Vecuronium
b. Atracurium
c. *d*-Tubocurarine
d. Pipecuronium

9. The neuromuscular drug of choice for endotracheal intubation is:
a. Vecuronium
b. Atracurium
c. d-Tubocurarine
d. Succinylcholine

10. For endotracheally intubated, paralyzed patients receiving mechanical ventilation, which of the following would help reduce the risk of aspiration?
a. Reduce the ventilator driving pressure
b. Raise the head of the bed
c. Have the patient supine with legs raised
d. Reduce the positive end-expiratory pressure (PEEP) to less than 5 cmH$_2$O

11. What should be administered to remove conscious awareness in a patient who has received a neuromuscular blocking agent?
    a. Heart medication
    b. Blood pressure medication
    c. Sedation
    d. Bronchodilator

12. What is the simplest means of monitoring the adequacy of neuromuscular blockade?
    a. Train of four
    b. Twitch monitoring
    c. Response to painful stimuli
    d. Direct observation of muscle activity

13. What would be the first indication that a nondepolarizing agent is reversing or wearing off?
    a. Eyelids move
    b. Extremities move
    c. The abdomen moves
    d. The patient swallows

14. During brief periods of paralysis, which of the following subjective assessments measures voluntary muscular functions?
    I. Hand grip strength
    II. The ability to lift the head off the bed for 5 seconds
    III. Heart rate returning to normal
    IV. Increase in $SpO_2$
        a. I and II only
        b. II and III only
        c. I, III, and IV only
        d. I, II, and IV only

You are called to the emergency department to assist in the care of patient who was in a motor vehicle accident. In the report you learn that he has pulmonary contusions and a flail chest. He does not respond to verbal commands and is combative. On the basis of his arterial blood gases and other physical findings you recommend that the patient be orally intubated. The patient is very restless.

1. Which neuromuscular blocking agent should you use to paralyze him? Why?

The patient is intubated and moved to the intensive care unit, where he is placed on mechanical ventilation. You learn from report by family members that he has other conditions including asthma. Over the next few hours the patient remains very restless. He is breathing asynchronously with the ventilator in spite of several changes made to the ventilator settings. You call the doctor and suggest a neuromuscular blocking agent.

2. Which type of blocking agent do you recommend? Why?

3. What type of blocking agent would you *not* want to use for this patient, and why?

4. Are there any other medications you would suggest for this patient receiving neuromuscular blocking agents?

5. While the patient is intubated and receiving mechanical ventilation, what can you do to reduce the incidence of nosocomial infection and aspiration while the patient is receiving a neuromuscular blocking agent?

The next day it is decided to begin reversing the neuromuscular blocking medication.

6. What would be the first response indicating the patient has begun breathing on his own?

# 19 Vasopressors, Inotropes, and Antiarrhythmic Agents

## CHAPTER OBJECTIVES

*After answering the following questions, the reader should be able to:*

1. List the various components that make up blood pressure
2. Understand the cardiovascular system and factors affecting blood pressure
3. Compare and contrast the mechanism of action of the different inotropes and vasopressors
4. Describe the various drug interactions that may occur with use of vasopressors and inotropes
5. Describe the normal conduction of the heart
6. Define the mechanism of action of digoxin
7. Define the nonpharmacologic methods of treating dysrhythmias
8. List the various routes by which to administer medications during cardiac arrest
9. List the benefits and disadvantages of using sodium bicarbonate therapy in the setting of cardiac arrest

## KEY TERMS AND DEFINITIONS

*Match the following definitions with their terms.*

1. _____ The presence of carbon dioxide aiding in the release and delivery of oxygen from hemoglobin

2. _____ The amount of blood that is ejected into the aorta and travels through the systemic circulation with every heartbeat

3. _____ The lowest pressure reached right before ventricular ejection

4. _____ Pressure that drives blood into the tissues, averaged over the entire cardiac cycle

5. _____ Cardiac medications that are classified, according to the Vaughan Williams classification system, according to their mechanism of action. In some instances they may present multiple mechanisms of action.

6. _____ Endogenous products that are secreted into the blood stream and travel to nerve endings to stimulate an excitatory response

7. _____ Link between atrial depolarization and ventricular depolarization

8. _____ Peak pressure reached during ventricular ejection

9. _____ An episode of ventricular fibrillation, pulseless ventricular tachycardia, pulseless electrical activity, or asystole

10. _____ An enzyme responsible for the breakdown of cyclic adenosine 3′,5′-monophosphate (cAMP)

a. Antiarrhythmics
b. Atrioventricular (AV) node
c. Bohr effect
d. Cardiac output
e. Catecholamines
f. Diastolic blood pressure (DBP)
g. Mean arterial pressure (MAP)
h. Phosphodiesterase
i. Sudden cardiac death (SCD)
j. Systolic blood pressure (SBP)

The cardiovascular system is a complex system that touches each tissue bed in the body. Without the appropriate blood flow, without the delivery of nutrients and oxygen and the removal of waste products, the organs of the body would not function properly. Tissue perfusion depends on three major factors: cardiac function, vascular tone, and vascular volume.

Cardiac function refers to cardiac output and ventricular contractility. Cardiac output, the amount of blood pumped by each ventricle of the heart per minute, is determined as the product of heart rate times stroke volume, or the amount of blood ejected from each ventricle per beat. Cardiac output is a major determinant of blood pressure. Ventricular contractility is influenced mainly by the volume of blood filling the ventricles (preload) and can be modified by inotropic drugs. A chronotropic effect increases the rate of contraction of the heart and an inotropic effect increases contractility of the heart.

Vascular tone (systemic vascular resistance) is regulated by the sympathetic nervous system and by circulating hormones. Local regulation also can be influenced by local oxygen levels and acid–base status. Vascular volume is the second major determinant of blood pressure. Vascular volume will have an impact on stroke volume and is regulated mainly by the kidneys.

These factors all interrelate to maintain stable tissue perfusion and proper cardiovascular function. When disease processes affect components of the cardiovascular system, abnormal conditions will occur. During these times pharmacological intervention is used to help maintain normal function.

Typical measurement of blood pressure is relative to a recurring cardiac cycle of atrial and ventricular contractions and relaxations. The cycle is divided into systolic and diastolic phases. The mean arterial pressure (MAP) is actually of greater significance than the SBP and the DBP. The mean arterial pressure signifies the pressure that drives blood into the tissues averaged over the entire cardiac cycle.

11. What is the cardiac output of a patient with a blood pressure of 120/70, a stroke volume of 70 ml/beat, and a heart rate of 80 beats/min?

12. Ventricular contractility is influenced mainly by the volume of blood filling the ventricles, called the

_____, and can be modified by inotropic drugs.

13. What are two determinants of arterial blood pressure?

a. _____

b. _____

14. What is the mean arterial blood pressure of a patient who has a blood pressure of 120/90?

15. What pressure helps reflect the amount of blood returning to the heart?

*List the normal pressures of each hemodynamic parameter. (Hint: Review Table 19-1.)*

16. Central venous pressure (CVP): _____

17. Pulmonary capillary wedge pressure (PCWP): _____

18. Cardiac output (CO): _____

19. Systemic vascular resistance (SVR): _____

*Given the following shock states, determine what will happen to the hemodynamic parameter.*

20. _____ Heart rate with hypovolemia/hemorrhagic shock      a. Increase
     b. Decrease

21. _____ CVP with hypovolemia/hemorrhagic shock

22. _____ CO with hypovolemia/hemorrhagic shock

23. _____ SVR with cardiogenic shock

24. _____ BP with septic shock

25. _____ PCWP with hypovolemic/hemorrhagic shock

26. _____ CO with septic shock

## AGENTS USED IN THE MANAGEMENT OF SHOCK

Agents used in the management of shock include catecholamines, inotropic agents, phosphodiesterase inhibitors, and cardiac glycosides.

### Catecholamines

27. Catecholamines such as norepinephrine (Levophed) and epinephrine (Adrenalin) cause _____ of the vasculature by affecting α receptors.

28. Dopamine (Inotropin) increases chronotropic and inotropic effects, leading to increased _____ output.

29. Vasopressin (Pitressin) may be used for _____ shock.

### Inotropic Agents

30. True or False: Dobutamine (Dobutrex) is indicated for short-term treatment of decompensated heart failure secondary to depressed contractility.

**Phosphodiesterase Inhibitors**

31. True or False: Phosphodiesterase inhibitors such as inamrinone (Inocor) increase myocardial contractility.

**Cardiac Glycosides**

32. Digoxin (Lanoxin), the only drug in the cardiac glycoside class, is used in the management of chronic

_____ _____.


## ELECTROPHYSIOLOGY OF THE MYOCARDIUM

The cardiac electrical conduction system is made up of specialized cells. The major components include the sinoatrial (SA) node, the AV node, the bundle of His, the ventricular bundle branches, and the Purkinje fibers.

The SA node is located in the right atrium near the superior vena cava. Its ability to elicit spontaneous impulses (automaticity), that is, depolarize, is normally more rapid than in any other area of the heart. This fact results in the SA node being the pacemaker of the heart. Heartbeats originating in the SA node are called sinus beats or a sinus rhythm. Although the depolarization wave will travel through each of the muscle cells of the atria, special conduction fibers (internodal pathways) connect the SA node to the AV node. A special fiber, Bachmann's bundle, also runs from the SA node to the left atrium.

The AV node is located in the inferior right atrium above the tricuspid valve. The bundle of His is a continuation of the AV node into the ventricular septum. Normally the AV node/bundle of His is considered to be the only electrical pathway from the atria to the ventricles, and it allows current to flow in only one direction.

The bundle branches are the continuation of the electrical system into the ventricular septum and into the ventricular walls. The terminal ends of the bundle branches are the Purkinje fibers. They infiltrate the myocardial muscle cells (arranged as a functional syncytium), which allows the impulse to travel over the entire heart muscle. In normal function, each time the SA node "fires," a heartbeat will occur. Heart rate can be affected by many factors including blood pressure, oxygen demand, body position, exercise, fever, and intrathoracic and intracranial pressure. Stimulation of the sympathetic nervous system will cause the heart rate to increase. Stimulation of the parasympathetic nervous system will cause a decrease in heart rate.

33. List the five major components of the heart's electrical conduction system:

   a. _____

   b. _____

   c. _____

   d. _____

   e. _____


## PHARMACOLOGY OF ANTIARRHYTHMICS

**Class IA**

Class I agents are membrane-stabilizing or local anesthetics that depress the fast inward current of sodium (phase 0). Examples include the following:

34. Quinidine (Quinaglute) is used to treat atrial _____ and _____.

35. Procainamide (Procanbid) is used to treat ventricular _____ and atrial arrhythmias.

**Class IB**

Class IB agents are often used and have less proarrhythmic potential compared with the class IA agents. The actions of class IB agents are limited to ventricular arrhythmias.

36. Lidocaine is used to control _____ arrhythmias such as premature ventricular contraction (PVCs), ventricular tachycardia, and ventricular fibrillation.

## Class II

Class II agents are β-adrenergic blocking agents. They block $\beta_1$ receptors in the heart to control dysrhythmias. Heart rate is reduced, AV conduction is prolonged, and contractile force is decreased. In the setting in which patients with airway disease are overly sensitive to the bronchoconstrictive effects of β blockers, esmolol may be a convenient selection. Because of esmolol's short half-life of ~10 minutes, one may titrate the dose to meet the patient's therapeutic and safety goals.

37. A side effect of class II agents in patients with airway disease is the potential for _____.

## Class III

Class III agents such as amiodarone (Cordarone) prolong the duration of phase 3 repolarization and therefore the effective refractory period (i.e., they prolong the action potential).

38. In general, class III agents are used to treat supraventricular arrhythmias and _____ arrhythmias.

## Class IV

Class IV agents manage supraventricular arrhythmias as well as ventricular rate control for atrial fibrillation.

39. Class IV drugs such as verapamil (Isoptin) and diltiazem (Cardizem) are called _____

_____ blockers.

## MANAGEMENT AND PHARMACOTHERAPY OF ADVANCED CARDIAC LIFE SUPPORT

*The following is a list of drugs used for advanced life support. Next to the drug give the indication for that drug.*

40. Epinephrine: _____

41. Vasopressin: _____

42. Atropine: _____

43. Sodium bicarbonate: _____

44. Magnesium sulfate: _____

*Answer the following questions.*

45. When would intraosseous needle placement be indicated?

46. List the drugs that can be administered via an endotracheal tube (ETT) if IV access is not available.

    a. _____

    b. _____

    c. _____

    d. _____

47. True or False: When medications are administered through the ETT, chest compressions should not cease.

48. True or False: Medications should be placed in the ETT through a catheter that extends beyond the tip of the ETT.

49. True or False: After medication insertion into the lung, 5–10 rapid ventilations with a hand-held resuscitation bag should take place.

50. True or False: Medications should be diluted with approximately 10 ml of normal saline when administering them through the ETT.

## NATIONAL BOARD OF RESPIRATORY CARE–TYPE QUESTIONS

1. Pressure that drives blood into the tissues, averaged over the entire cardiac cycle, is:
   a. Systolic pressure
   b. Systemic vascular pressure
   c. Mean arterial pressure
   d. Diastolic pressure

2. A patient has a cardiac output of 5.6 L/min and a heart rate of 80 beats/min. What is the stroke volume?
   a. 100 ml/beat
   b. 90 ml/beat
   c. 80 ml/beat
   d. 70 ml/beat

3. Which of the following pressures reflects the amount of blood returning to the heart?
   a. Central venous pressure
   b. Mean arterial pressure
   c. Pulmonary artery pressure
   d. Pulmonary capillary wedge pressure

4. The normal cardiac output in an adult is:
   a. 8–10 L/min
   b. 5–7 L/min
   c. 1–3 L/min
   d. 10–12 L/min

5. Agents used in the management of shock include:
   I. Catecholamines
   II. Inotropes
   III. Phosphodiesterase inhibitors
   IV. Cardiac glycosides
      a. I and II only
      b. II and III only
      c. I and IV only
      d. I, II, III, and IV

6. Norepinephrine and epinephrine are:
   a. Catecholamines
   b. Inotropes
   c. Phosphodiesterase inhibitors
   d. Cardiac glycosides

7. Which of the following is an inotopic agent that is indicated for short-term treatment of decompensated heart failure secondary to depressed contractility?
   a. Dopamine (Inotropin)
   b. Vasopressin (Pitressin)
   c. Dobutamine (Dobutrex)
   d. Digoxin (Lanoxin)

8. The only cardiac glycoside that is used in the management of chronic heart failure is:
   a. Dopamine
   b. Digoxin
   c. Dobutamine
   d. Epinephrine

Chapter 19 Vasopressors, Inotropes, and Antiarrhythmic Agents

9. Which of the following is *not* a major component of the heart's electrical conduction system?
   a. SA node
   b. AV node
   c. Bundle of His
   d. Mitral valve

10. Which of the following drugs is in class IB and is used to control arrhythmias such as PVCs, ventricular tachycardia, and ventricular fibrillation?
    a. Quinidine
    b. Procainamide
    c. Lidocaine
    d. Propranolol

11. This drug is used increase arterial blood pH above 7.2. Adequate ventilation must be present to remove the carbon dioxide produced, otherwise intracellular pH will begin to decline.
    a. Atropine
    b. Vasopressin
    c. Magnesium sulfate
    d. Sodium bicarbonate

12. If IV access is not available in a patient with cardiac arrest, which of the following drugs can be administered via an endotracheal tube (ETT)?
    I. Lidocaine
    II. Epinephrine
    III. Atropine
    IV. Naloxone
       a. I and II only
       b. II and III only
       c. I, II, and IV only
       d. I, II, III, and IV

13. Which of the following statements is *false* regarding the administration of medications through the ETT of a patient in cardiac arrest?
    a. Medications should be placed in the ETT through a catheter that extends beyond the tip of the ETT.
    b. After medication insertion into the lung, 5–10 rapid ventilations with a hand-held resuscitation bag should take place.
    c. Chest compressions should continue as drugs are administered through the ETT.
    d. Medications should be diluted with approximately 10 ml of normal saline when administering them via the ETT.

14. Which of the following are determinants of blood pressure?
    I. Vascular volume
    II. Preload
    III. Central venous pressure
    IV. Systemic vascular resistance
       a. II and III only
       b. I and IV only
       c. II, III, and IV only
       d. I, II, III, and IV

15. What is the mean arterial pressure of a patient with a blood pressure of 110/80?
    a. 60 mmHg
    b. 85 mmHg
    c. 90 mmHg
    d. 100 mmHg

A 19-year-old is brought into the emergency department by ambulance, following an automobile accident. The paramedics tell you she has lost a lot of blood. She is intubated and being ventilated with a hand-held resuscitation bag with 100% oxygen. She has IV access.

1. On the basis of this information, what shock state would you treat her for?

2. How would you expect the following hemodynamic parameters to be altered for this patient, based on your answer to question 1? (And make an educated guess as to what these values would be as a result of her condition.)

    a. BP: _____

    b. Heart rate: _____

    c. CVP: _____

    d. CO: _____

    e. SVR: _____

The patient begins to have numerous PVCs. The doctor orders lidocaine. The IV access is no longer available and because of her low blood pressure, no IV access can be found.

3. What would you recommend?

IV access has been reestablished and a CVP catheter has been inserted. The patient has been treated with various drugs and volume and now her hemodynamic parameters are as follows:
    Heart rate: 87 beats/min
    CVP: 9 mmHg
    Blood pressure: 110/78

4. How would you evaluate her hemodynamic profile?

# Drugs Affecting Circulation: Antihypertensives, Antianginals, Antithrombotics

## CHAPTER OBJECTIVES

*After answering the following questions, the reader should be able to:*

1. Categorize the stages of normal to high blood pressure
2. Define a hypertensive crisis
3. Compare and contrast the clinical pharmacology among the agents used for hypertensive pharmacotherapy
4. Describe the mechanism of action of the angiotensin-converting enzyme inhibitors, calcium channel blockers, and β blockers
5. Compare and contrast the clinical pharmacology of spironolactone and eplerenone
6. List antihypertensive relevant drug-drug interactions, and plausible mechanisms
7. Describe the formation and elimination of an acute coronary thrombus
8. List the agents in each of the following antithrombotic classes: anticoagulants, antiplatelets, and thrombolytics
9. Describe the mechanism of action of heparin
10. List the laboratory parameters that may be used to monitor for the effect of heparin, low molecular weight heparin, and direct thrombin inhibitors
11. Compare and contrast the clinical pharmacology of aspirin, clopidogrel, ticlopidine, and dipyridamole
12. Describe the indication and mechanism of action of the glycoprotein IIb/IIIa inhibitors
13. Describe the formation and elimination of an acute coronary thrombus
14. List the indications of the thrombolytics

## KEY TERMS AND DEFINITIONS

*Match the following definitions with their terms.*

1. _____ Damage to the heart and the blood vessels or circulation, including the brain, kidney, and the eye

2. _____ A maximal dose of a drug beyond which it no longer exerts a therapeutic effect; however, its toxicologic effect does increase

3. _____ The volume of water filtered from the plasma by the kidney via the glomerular capillary walls into Bowman capsules per unit time; considered to be 90% of creatinine clearance, and equivalent to insulin clearance

4. _____ When a neurotransmitter or hormone is replaced by a different neurotransmitter or hormone, which can be weaker or inert

5. _____ Human biologic variations of rhythm within a 24-hour cycle

6. _____ Treatment of disease by drug therapy

a. Antithrombotic
b. Arterial blood pressure
c. Cardiovascular disease (CVD)
d. Chronotropic
e. Circadian rhythm
f. Creatinine clearance
g. D-dimers
h. Dose-ceiling effect
i. Drug substrate
j. Fibrinogen degradation products (FDPs)
k. Glomerular filtration rate (GFR)
l. Hypertensive emergency
m. Hypertensive urgency
n. Inotrope
o. Intrinsic sympathomimetic activity
p. Pharmacotherapy
q. Renin
r. Substitute neurotransmitters

7._____ A drug influencing the contractility of a muscle (i.e., the heart)

8. _____ Influencing the rate of rhythmic movements (i.e., the heartbeat)

9. _____ Drugs, such as anticoagulants, anti-platelets, and thrombolytics, that prevent or break up blood clots in such conditions as thrombosis or embolism

10. _____ Measurement of the renal clearance of endogenous creatinine per unit time; considered to be an estimate of the glomerular filtration rate (GFR); overesti-mates GFR by 10%-15%; used for drug-dosing guidelines

11. _____ Defined hemodynamically as the product of cardiac output (heart rate × stroke volume) and total peripheral resistance

12. _____ Covalently cross-linked degradation fragments of the cross-linked fibrin poly-mer during plasmin-mediated fibrinolysis; the level increases after the onset of fibri-nolysis, and allows for the identification of the presence of fibrinolysis

13. _____ An enzyme, also known as angiotensino-genase, that is released by the kidney in response to a lack of renal blood flow, and responsible for converting angiotensinogen into angiotensin I

14. _____ Blood pressures above 180/120 mmHg when the elevation of blood pressure is accompanied by acute, chronic, or progressing target organ injury

15. _____ The drug acted on or induced or inhibited (during a drug–drug interaction); the reactant

16. _____ Blood pressures above 180/120 mmHg without signs or symptoms of acute target organ complications

17. _____ Small peptides that result following the action of plasmin on fibrinogen and fibrin in the fibrinolytic process. They are anti-coagulant substances that can cause bleeding if fibrinolysis becomes uncon-trolled and excessive

18. _____ A drug that activates and blocks adrener-gic receptors, producing a net stimulatory effect on the sympathetic nervous system

## EPIDEMIOLOGY AND ETIOLOGY OF HYPERTENSION

Hypertension is defined as a blood pressure more than 140/90 mmHg that has been documented on separate days. It affects more than 60 million Americans. The majority of cases are of unknown etiology and are termed primary or essential hypertension. A diastolic pressure more than 120 mmHg with acute organ injury is a hypertensive emergency requiring immediate blood pressure reduction.

19. Optimal blood pressure for adults 18 years of age or greater is a systolic pressure less than

    _____ and a diastolic pressure less than _____.

20. True or False: Hypertension occurs more frequently in males than females and in more blacks than whites.

21. A patient with blood pressure above 180/120 mmHg is considered to be in a(n) _____

    _____.


## HYPERTENSION PHARMACOTHERAPY

### Angiotensin-converting Enzyme Inhibitors

Angiotensin-converting enzyme (ACE) inhibitors suppress the renin–angiotensin–aldosterone system. Renin, released from the kidneys, stimulates the production of angiotensin I in the plasma. In the lungs, angiotensin I is converted to angiotensin II by angiotensin-converting enzyme. Angiotensin II is a powerful vasoconstrictor. Angiotensin II also stimulates aldosterone secretion, which increases fluid retention and stimulates release of catecholamines. By blocking the action of ACE, angiotensin II is not produced and blood pressure will drop. ACE inhibitors (ACEIs) also block the breakdown of bradykinin and other vasodilators; this contributes to decreasing blood pressure as well. ACE inhibitors are most effective in normal to high renin hypertension. The most common side effects of ACE inhibitors are a dry cough and a skin rash. ACE inhibitors should not be used during pregnancy because of the potential of fetal morbidity.

22. ACEIs act primarily through suppression of the _____–_____–

    _____ system.

23. List two hemodynamic effects of ACEIs.

    a. _____

    b. _____


### Angiotensin II Receptor Blockers

Several pathways other than the ACE and renin pathway produce angiotensin II. Therefore ACE inhibitors do not completely block angiotensin II production. Angiotensin II receptor blockers prevent the effects of angiotensin II at receptors found on vascular smooth muscle and other organs. Their antihypertensive effect is similar to that of the ACE inhibitors.

### Calcium Channel Blockers

Cellular influx of calcium from extracellular fluid is required for vascular smooth muscle contraction. Calcium channel blockers decrease calcium influx, thus helping to prevent smooth muscle contraction and resultant hypertension.

24. True or False: Angiotensin II receptor blockers (ARBs) are indicated for hypertension and can be used for the treatment of heart failure.

25. What are three indications for the calcium channel blocker (CCB) verapamil?

    a. _____

    b. _____

    c. _____

26. Verapamil has negative chronotropic effects and negative inotropic effects. What does this mean?

27. True or False: The majority of myocardial infarctions (MIs), strokes, dysrhythmias, and venous thromboembolic events occur in the evening hours, in concert with the circadian blood pressure peaks.

## β BLOCKERS

The β blockers have multiple pathways of effect that can reduce blood pressure. These include renin blockade, resulting in decreased angiotensin II production; blockade of myocardial β receptors, resulting in decreased cardiac output; blockade of central nervous system (CNS) β receptors, leading to decreased sympathetic output; and blockade of peripheral β receptors, resulting in decreased norepinephrine concentrations. β Blockers may cause pulmonary side effects including bronchospasm and exacerbation of asthma. Patients receiving β blockers should be monitored closely because of the multiple side effects of these drugs.

28. List six symptoms of β-blocker–induced pulmonary dysfunction:

a. _____

b. _____

c. _____

d. _____

e. _____

f. _____

### Diuretics

Diuretics work in the kidney to increase water excretion. Increased excretion of water will reduce fluid volume and aid in reducing blood pressure. There are five classes of diuretics but only two, the potassium-sparing and thiazide diuretics, are routinely used to lower blood pressure. Most diuretics not only cause excess water excretion but also cause electrolyte loss. The potassium-sparing diuretics help retain body potassium. They are weak antihypertensives but, when used with other diuretics, provide a beneficial effect. Use of the thiazide diuretics results in mild diuresis, but their main antihypertensive activity is associated with their ability to cause vasodilation.

29. Of the five classes of diuretics which two are used to manage hypertension?

a. _____

b. _____

### Aldosterone Antagonists

Spironolactone (Aldactone) and eplerenone (Inspra) are aldosterone antagonists that exert their effect on the late distal tubule and collecting duct. Spironolactone is used a weak diuretic, primarily for its aldosterone antagonist effects. Spironolactone is indicated for hypertension and heart failure. Eplerenone is indicated for heart failure subsequent to MI and hypertension.

### Centrally Acting Adrenergic Agents: α2 Agonists

Centrally acting adrenergic α2 agonists decrease sympathetic nerve stimulation from the CNS. Because of their significant side effects, the α2 agonists are not used as first-line agents even though they are potent antihypertensives.

**194**

$\alpha_2$ Agonists lower blood pressure by affecting both cardiac output and peripheral resistance; they are negative inotropes and chronotropes. The $\alpha_2$ agonists are not recommended for noncompliant patients and should never be withdrawn abruptly because of the risk of either rebound hypertension or overshoot hypertension.

### $\alpha_1$-Adrenergic Antagonists

$\alpha_1$-Adrenergic antagonists block the postsynaptic $\alpha_1$ receptors, resulting in both arterial and venous dilation. Total peripheral resistance is reduced through both arterial and venous dilation; thus these agents decrease both preload and afterload. These agents have significant side effects. One drug, doxazosin, has been shown to have a higher morbidity rate than other antihypertensives. They are not recommended as first-line agents.

30. How do $\alpha_2$ agonists lower blood pressure?

### Antiadrenergic Agents

The antiadrenergic antihypertensive agents are reserpine, guanethidine (Ismelin), and guanadrel (Hylorel). All three of these agents are second-line antihypertensives.

### Vasodilators

The two common vasodilators used in the management of hypertension are hydralazine (Apresoline) and minoxidil (Rogaine, Loniten). Because of their adverse effects profile the vasodilators are second-line antihypertensive agents. These agents reduce total peripheral resistance by a direct action on vascular smooth muscle, increasing intracellular concentrations of cyclic guanosine monophosphate (cGMP).

31. How does the antihypertensive drug hydralazine (Apresoline) reduce total peripheral resistance to reduce blood pressure?

### EPIDEMIOLOGY, ETIOLOGY, AND PATHOPHYSIOLOGY OF ANGINA

Angina pectoris (chest pain) is the most common symptom of myocardial ischemia. Ischemia results when blood flow and oxygen delivery do not meet myocardial oxygen demand. Angina may present as chest tightness, pressure, or a burning sensation (indigestion) and may radiate to the left shoulder and jaw. Factors that increase myocardial oxygen demand include increased heart rate, increased systolic wall force or tension, and increased contractility. Factors that decrease myocardial oxygen supply include a decrease in the concentration of oxygen (e.g., anemia), a decrease in coronary blood flow (e.g., thrombus), and an inability of the myocardium to extract oxygen from the blood. Drugs used to treat angina include nitrates, $\beta$ blockers, calcium antagonists, and ranolazine (Ranexa). All patients with angina should receive aspirin for prophylaxis of an MI.

32. List three symptoms exhibited by a patient experiencing angina:

    a. _____

    b. _____

    c. _____

## Nitrates

Nitrates can be administered by several routes. Nitroglycerin, a commonly used nitrate, is a sublingual agent used for acute angina relief. Nitroglycerin reduces myocardial oxygen demand by causing venodilation of coronary arteries and collaterals, resulting in decreased end-diastolic pressures. Sublingual nitroglycerin has an onset of action of minutes and duration of action of 30 minutes. Sublingual nitroglycerin should be administered every 5 minutes until relief is obtained. If no pain relief is achieved after three doses in 15 minutes, seek emergency care. Side effects are minimal and include increased heart rate, palpitations, headache, and flushing of the skin. Tolerance may occur with prolonged use. Open containers should be discarded after 6 months.

33. How is anginal pain relieved with nitrates such as nitroglycerin?

34. How is nitroglycerin administered for acute relief of anginal pain?

35. How often should nitroglycerin be administered for relief of anginal pain?

## Ranolazine

Ranolazine is indicated for the treatment of chronic angina patients who have not achieved an adequate response with other antianginal drugs. Ranolazine increase exercise tolerance reduces angina frequency, and the need for emergent nitroglycerin interventions. Ranolazine is an extended-release tablet given twice a day. Adverse reactions observed with ranolazine include dizziness, palpitations, headache, constipation, nausea, abdominal pain, and peripheral edema.

36. What is the indication for ranolazine?

## ANTITHROMBOTIC AGENTS

Antithrombotics are agents that prevent or break up blood clots in such conditions as thrombosis or embolism. Clot formation occurs at sites of injury. After an injury, platelet attraction and aggregation are the first steps in clot formation. Fibrinogen binding and formation of fibrin are the final steps in clot formation. Normally the body maintains a state of equilibrium between clot formation and clot breakdown. In abnormal states, antithrombotic therapy should be instituted. Antithrombotics are divided into three categories: antiplatelet agents (aspirin) inhibit the action of platelets; anticoagulants (heparin and warfarin) prevent the formation of fibrin clots; and thrombolytics (urokinase) break down fibrin clots.

**196**

## Anticoagulant Agents

### Heparin

Heparin is commonly used in the treatment and prevention of venous thromboembolism and pulmonary embolism. The activated partial thromboplastin time (APTT) is used to monitor high molecular weight heparin effects and should be maintained at 2 to 2.5 times the control value. The onset of action of heparin is within 6 hours after the initiation of a continuous infusion. The activated partial thromboplastin time (aPTT) is used to monitor heparin's effects. Protamine sulfate is the antidote for heparin and should be administered by slow intravenous infusion over at least 1 to 3 minutes to prevent hypotension, bradycardia, and dyspnea.

### Direct Thrombin Inhibitors

There are four commercially available highly specific direct thrombin inhibitors (DTIs). Desirudin (Iprivask) is indicated for deep vein thrombosis prophylaxis, and bivalirudin (Angiomax) is indicated for unstable angina. Argatroban and lepirudin (Refludan) are indicated for prophylaxis or treatment of thrombosis in patients with heparin-induced thrombocytopenia type 2 (HIT-2) and are used for anticoagulation against thromboembolic conditions in patients with or at risk for HIT-2.

### Warfarin (Coumadin)

Warfarin (Coumadin) is an oral anticoagulant indicated for the prophylaxis and treatment of venous thrombosis, pulmonary embolism, and thromboembolic complications associated with atrial fibrillation and cardiac valve replacement, and as an adjunct in the treatment of coronary occlusion. Warfarin is also used to reduce the risk of death, reinfarction, and thromboembolic events such as stroke or systemic embolization after MI. It has a longer time for onset and a longer duration of action than heparin. When a patient is switched from heparin therapy to warfarin therapy, heparin should not be immediately discontinued. Heparin therapy should continue until warfarin has taken effect. The complete antithrombotic effects of warfarin may not occur until 5 to 7 days after initiation of therapy. It is suggested that the international normalized ratio (INR) be used for monitoring warfarin therapy and not prothrombin time (PT). The INR should be maintained at two to three times the control value. Vitamin K is an antidote for warfarin therapy. Hemorrhage is the most common adverse effect.

37. What are two indications for heparin therapy?

    a. _____

    b. _____

38. True or False: As compared with heparin, warfarin has a longer time for onset and longer duration.

## Antiplatelet Agents

### Aspirin

Aspirin's antithrombotic indications include reducing the risk of thrombosis, such as in the primary and secondary prevention of nonfatal or fatal MI in patients with/or without a previous MI or unstable angina, and preventing recurrent transient ischemic attacks or stroke. High doses of aspirin are used for its analgesic, antiinflammatory, and antipyretic effects and low doses of aspirin are used for its antithrombotic indications. Aspirin, especially at high doses, can induce or exacerbate asthma and dyspnea in patients with chronic obstructive pulmonary disease (COPD).

### Dipyridamole (Persantine)

Dipyridamole (Persantine) is a vasodilator and platelet adhesion inhibitor. Dipyridamole is only indicated as an adjunct to warfarin in the prevention of postoperative thromboembolic complications of cardiac valve replacement.

### Clopidogrel (Plavix)

Clopidogrel is a prodrug thienopyridine derivative platelet aggregation inhibitor. It interferes with platelet membrane function by inhibiting adenosine diphosphate (ADP)-induced platelet–fibrinogen binding and subsequent platelet–platelet interactions. The indications for clopidogrel include the reduction of atherosclerotic events in patients with a history of MI, stroke, or peripheral arteriolar disease, and for an acute coronary syndrome regardless of whether a patient will be managed medically or with percutaneous coronary intervention, or coronary artery bypass graft.

### Ticlopidine (Ticlid)

Ticlopidine is a platelet aggregation inhibitor that interferes with platelet membrane function by inhibiting ADP-induced platelet–fibrinogen binding and subsequent platelet–platelet interactions. Ticlopidine is indicated for stroke.

## Cilostazol (Pletal) and Pentoxifylline

Cilostazol is a quinolinone derivative that selectively and reversibly inhibits cellular phosphodiesterase III by increasing the levels of cAMP, resulting in vasodilation and inhibition of platelet aggregation.

## Glycoprotein IIb/IIIa Inhibitors

The glycoprotein (GP) IIb/IIIa inhibitors are indicated for the treatment of patients with acute coronary syndromes—unstable angina or non–ST-elevation acute MI, including patients who are medically managed and those undergoing percutaneous coronary intervention (PCI). The most common adverse effect reported during therapy was bleeding.

39. What is a concern when aspirin is given at high doses to asthma and COPD patients?

40. True or False: One indication for the antiplatelet agent Plavix is the reduction of atherosclerotic events in patients with a history of MI, stroke, or peripheral arteriolar disease.

## Thrombolytics

Thrombolytics can restore blood flow to blocked areas by dissolving the clot. Two critical areas for use include the brain and coronary artery circulation. Thrombolytics reduce the incidence of heart failure and death associated with an acute MI and restore coronary blood flow by dissolving the thrombus, thus limiting the extent of ischemia and necrosis. Therapy should be instituted as soon as possible after the onset of symptoms. It is recommended that therapy be given within 1 hour in stroke patients and in less than 6 hours for patients with heart attacks. Quick response helps to prevent extensive tissue ischemia and necrosis. Examples of these drugs include streptokinase, alteplase, reteplase, and tenecteplase. The most common adverse effect associated with these agents is major and minor bleeding.

41. True or False: It is recommended that thrombolytics therapy be given within 1 hour in stroke patients and in less than 6 hours for patients with heart attacks.

## NATIONAL BOARD OF RESPIRATORY CARE–TYPE QUESTIONS

1. Which of the following is optimal blood pressure for adults 18 years of age or greater?
   a. <120/<80
   b. >135/>85
   c. >140/>90
   d. <150/>70

2. Which of the statements is *false* regarding hypertension in adults?
   a. Hypertension occurs more frequently in males.
   b. Hypertension occurs more frequently in females.
   c. Hypertension occurs more blacks.
   d. Hypertension occurs less in whites.

3. Which of the following patients is in a hypertensive crisis?
   a. A patient with a blood pressure of 80/60
   b. A patient with a blood pressure 100/80
   c. A patient with a very low diastolic pressure, <30 mmHg
   d. A patient with blood pressure above 180/120 mmHg

4. Which of the following is *not* a hemodynamic effect of ACEIs?
   a. A reduction in peripheral arterial resistance
   b. An increase in cardiac output
   c. An increase in heart rate
   d. An increase in renal blood flow and unchanged glomerular filtration rate (GFR)

5. Which of the following is *not* an indication for calcium channel blockers such as verapamil?
    I. Angina
    II. Arrhythmias
    III. Hypertension
    IV. Low blood pressure
        a. I and II only
        b. II and III only
        c. I, II, and III only
        d. II, II, and IV only

6. The majority of MIs, strokes, dysrhythmias, and venous thromboembolic events occur in the

    _____ _____, in concert with the circadian blood pressure peaks.
        a. Morning hours
        b. Afternoon hours
        c. Evening hours
        d. Relaxation hours

7. Which of the following pulmonary symptoms may occur with the administration of β blockers?
    I. Bronchospasm
    II. Wheezing
    III. Dyspnea
    IV. Cough
        a. I and II only
        b. II and III only
        c. II, III, and IV only
        d. I, II, III, and IV

8. Of the five classes of diuretics which are used to manage hypertension?
    I. Thiazides
    II. Potassium-sparing agents
    III. Adrenergic agents
    IV. Antiadrenergic agents
        a. I and II only
        b. II and III only
        c. III and IV only
        d. I and IV only

9. How do $\alpha_2$ agonists lower blood pressure?
    a. By affecting both cardiac output and glomerular filtration rate
    b. By increasing peripheral vascular resistance
    c. By their negative inotropic and chronotropic effects
    d. By increasing the preload and afterload of the heart

10. Which of the following symptoms are exhibited by a patient experiencing angina?
    I. Chest tightness
    II. Pressure
    III. Burning sensation (indigestion)
    IV. Pain radiating to left shoulder and jaw
        a. I and II only
        b. II and III only
        c. I, III, and IV only
        d. I, II, III, and IV

11. How is anginal pain relieved with nitrates such as nitroglycerin?
    a. Reduction in cardiac output
    b. Vasodilation of coronary arteries
    c. Peripheral vascular vasodilation
    d. Reduction in platelet adherence to peripheral vasculature

12. A patient with anginal pain was administered a nitroglycerin tablet 5 minutes ago. There is no relief from the pain. What would you recommend?
    a. Seek emergency care
    b. Wait 30 minutes before taking another nitroglycerin tablet
    c. Take another nitroglycerin tablet immediately
    d. Take two nitroglycerin tablets immediately

13. Which of the following is an indication for heparin therapy?
    I. Prevention of venous thromboembolism
    II. Prevention of coronary artery vasoconstriction
    III. Prevention of platelet adhesion
    IV. Prevention of pulmonary vascular vasoconstriction
        a. I only
        b. IV only
        c. II and III only
        d. II, III, and IV only

14. It is recommended that thrombolytics therapy be administered how long after a stroke has occurred?
    a. Less than 6 hours
    b. Less than 12 hours
    c. No earlier than 3 hours
    d. Within 1 hour

15. What is a concern when aspirin is given at high doses to asthma patients?
    a. It can induce severe bleeding from the GI tract
    b. It can exacerbate asthma symptoms
    c. Minor bleeding may occur within the pulmonary tract
    d. It can increase the changes of stroke

Mrs. A is a 69-year-old with a history of hypertension and angina. She was treated in the hospital 4 months ago for angina with nitrates and β blockers. She was sent home with nitroglycerin tablets and told to take one aspirin a day. This was the only episode of angina and she has not had angina since then. Early one morning Mrs. A got out of bed and was washing her face. Suddenly she began feeling light-headed with some mild chest discomfort. She turned to her husband and said, "I think I'm having another attack." Mr. A asks his wife how she feels.

1. On the basis of her history, what do you think are Mrs. A's symptoms?

2. Mr. A goes to the medicine cabinet to get nitroglycerin pills. He notices that the pills are 4 months old. Can he still use these pills?

3. Mrs. A puts a nitroglycerin pill under her tongue. How long before she should start feeling relief?

4. It has been 5 minutes since taking the first nitroglycerin pill and Mrs. A has felt no relief from her symptoms. What would you recommend?

5. It has now been 15 minutes and Mr. A has given his wife three nitroglycerin pills, There has been no relief. What should Mr. A do now?

# 21 Diuretic Agents

## CHAPTER OBJECTIVES

*After answering the following questions, the reader should be able to:*

1. Define *diuretics*
2. Describe renal function, filtration, reabsorption, and acid–base balance
3. List and describe the various groups of diuretics
4. List some of the indications for diuretic therapy
5. List the most common adverse reactions associated with the use of diuretics
6. Describe special situations related to diuretic therapy

## KEY TERMS AND DEFINITIONS

*Match the following definitions with their terms.*

1. _____ Swelling due to an abnormal accumulation of fluid in intercellular spaces of the body

2. _____ Abnormally decreased volume of blood circulating in the body

3. _____ The microscopic functional unit of the kidney responsible for filtering and maintaining fluid balance. Each kidney is made of approximately 2 million of these

4. _____ Inadequacy of the heart as a pump failing to maintain adequacy of blood circulation, resulting in congestion and tissue edema

5. _____ Amount of urine produced in 24 hours. Normal urine output averages 30 to 60 ml/hr

6. _____ The return to the blood of most of the water, sodium, amino acids, and sugar that were removed during filtration; occurs mainly in the proximal tubule of the nephron

7. _____ The mechanism by which the hydrostatic pressure forces fluid out of the glomerular capillary into the renal ducts

8. _____ Renal lithiasis in which calcium deposits form in the renal parenchyma and result in reduced kidney function and the presence of blood in the urine

a. Congestive heart failure (CHF)
b. Edema
c. Glomerular filtration
d. Hypovolemia
e. Nephrocalcinosis
f. Nephron
g. Ototoxicity
h. Reabsorption
i. Synergistic effect
j. Urine output

9. _____ Damage of the ear, specifically the cochlea or auditory nerve and sometimes the vestibulum, by a toxin

10. _____ Situation where the effect of two chemicals on an organism is greater than the effect of each chemical individually

## RENAL STRUCTURE AND FUNCTION

The urinary system is one of four excretory pathways of the body including the large intestines, the skin, and the lungs. The basic functions of the renal system are to regulate body water, to maintain electrolyte balance including acid–base balance, and to eliminate waste products (urea, etc.). The renal system is composed of two kidneys, two ureters, the bladder, urethra, and associated blood flow, lymph vessels, and nerves. The kidneys are located below the diaphragm in the posterior aspect of the abdominal cavity known as the retroperitoneal space. The functional units of the kidney are called nephrons, with each kidney containing approximately 1 million units. In kidney disease 75% of the nephrons may be compromised before evidence of disease. Urine formed by the nephrons collects in the ureters, which drain into the bladder. Urine is excreted from the body through the urethra. Approximately 22% of cardiac output (1.1 L/min in a 70-kg person) flows through the kidneys.

The kidney receives blood flow from the renal artery. Blood flow to the nephron arrives through the afferent arteriole, which forms a capillary tuft called the glomerulus. Blood flow from the glomerulus again forms a vessel, this one called the efferent arteriole. This vessel expands into a capillary network that has a close association with the nephron's tubules, loop of Henle, and collecting duct. Finally, the blood flows into veins that collect in the renal vein (see Figure 21-1 in the textbook).

The glomerulus is made up of very leaky capillaries and is located inside Bowman's capsule, the beginning of the proximal tubule in the nephrons. It is here that blood filtration takes place (fluid moves from the blood vessel into the kidney tubule) at the rate of 130 ml/min. This filtrate is cell and protein free but is otherwise similar to blood plasma. Blood pressure and glomerular capillary blood flow influence the glomerular filtration rate. Tubular reabsorption (movement of substance from the renal tubule back into the blood stream) is the next step in regulating blood volume and composition. Passage of the filtrate through the proximal convoluted tubules, loop of Henle, distal convoluted tubules, and collecting ducts allows modification of the filtrate. Ninety-nine percent of the filtrate is normally reabsorbed into the blood stream along with select molecules and ions. The third step in urine formation is the process of secretion (movement of substance from the blood into the tubules). Secretion occurs as the fluid moves through the nephron, modifying the tubular fluid and ultimately urine. With 99% reabsorption of glomerular filtrate, urine formation occurs at approximately 1 ml/min.

Urine output is regulated by several mechanisms. Antidiuretic hormone (ADH), or vasopressin, is a hormone secreted by the posterior pituitary gland. Increased production results in increased renal reabsorption of water and decreased urine output. Aldosterone is a hormone secreted by the adrenal cortex. Increased blood levels increase renal reabsorption of water and decrease urine output. Stimulation of the renin–angiotensin system also results in water retention and decreased urine output. Atrial natriuretic peptide (ANP) is a secretory granule with vasoactive properties. It is released by the right atrium in response to increased heart filling pressures (increased preload, increased atrial stretch). Increased blood levels of ANP cause natriuresis (sodium excretion), increased glomerular filtration, and inhibition of the renin–angiotensin aldosterone system and result in increased urine output. Review Box 21-1 in the textbook for ions that are filtered and exchanged in the kidneys.

11. The functional units of the kidney are called _____, with each kidney containing approximately 1 million units.

12. Blood pressure and glomerular capillary blood flow influence the _____

_____ _____.

13. The right atrium releases _____ _____

_____ in response to increased heart filling pressures (increased preload, increased atrial stretch).

14. _____ _____, or vasopressin, is a hormone secreted by the posterior pituitary gland. Increased production results in increased renal reabsorption of water and decreased urine output.

15. Stimulation of the _____–_____ _____ also results in water retention and decreased urine output.

16. _____ or _____ will force Na$^+$ exchange for H$^+$, producing metabolic alkalosis.

## DIURETIC GROUPS

The main purpose of diuretics is to increase urine output, thus removing excess fluid from the body. Most diuretics work by blocking sodium reabsorption in the tubules, and where sodium goes, so goes water. There are five general classifications of diuretics, each having its effect at a specific site in the nephron.

### Osmotic Diuretics

Osmotic diuretics are filtered out of the blood at the glomerulus, but they are not reabsorbed. They block the reabsorption of sodium, chloride, and water in the proximal tubule and descending loop of Henle. In the distal tubule, sodium is exchanged for potassium, thus creating hypokalemia and only mild diuresis. Mannitol is the most commonly used osmotic diuretic. Being a large molecule, mannitol also is useful for decreasing cerebral edema because it does not cross the blood–brain barrier.

17. One common use of osmotic diuretics is to treat _____ _____.

18. Osmotic substances are potent diuretics that lead to increased excretion of _____ and

_____.

### Carbonic Anhydrase Inhibitors

Carbonic anhydrase (CA) is an intracellular enzyme found in red blood cells, renal tubular cells, and in the eye. CA increases the rate of bicarbonate hydration. Normally bicarbonate and sodium are reabsorbed into the blood. Carbonic anhydrase inhibitors (CAIs) work within the proximal tubule cells, inhibiting the reabsorption of bicarbonate and sodium. It is only a weak diuretic because some sodium and water are reabsorbed downstream in the loop of Henle. CAIs have the potential to cause metabolic acidosis because bicarbonate is not reabsorbed. Acetazolamide (Diamox) is a CAI that has some potential use in patients with glaucoma, metabolic alkalosis, or altitude sickness. In glaucoma, CAIs will decrease intraocular pressure. In metabolic alkalosis, use of CAIs will decrease bicarbonate levels, leading to a normalization of pH. CAIs have been used to prevent altitude sickness. Although the exact mechanism of action is unknown, respiratory stimulation created by a mild metabolic acidosis is one possible answer.

19. Diamox, a CAI, is used to treat _____ _____ because it will decrease bicarbonate levels, leading to normalize pH.

### Loop Diuretics

Loop diuretics inhibit chloride, sodium, and water reabsorption in the ascending loop of Henle. They are the most potent diuretics because they can virtually block reabsorption at this site. Furosemide (Lasix) is a commonly used loop diuretic and is the first line of defense for creatinine clearance values < 40 ml/min. IV-delivered loop diuretics also have an acute but short-lived vasodilatory effect manifested by decreased pulmonary capillary wedge pressure (PCWP), blood pressure, and systemic vascular resistance. In some patients loop diuretics cause stimulation of the sympathetic nervous system, resulting in increased afterload and decreased cardiac function. This effect also is short lived.

20. Patients receiving osmotic diuretics should have their _____ levels monitored for hypokalemia.

21. Loop diuretics are administered to patients with pulmonary edema to cause _____.

22. Apart from their diuretic effects, loop diuretics may cause an acute _____ effect.

23. After administration of a loop diuretic, diuresis should take place within _____ minutes. If it doesn't the dose should be _____.

## Thiazide Diuretics

Thiazide diuretics block sodium, chloride, and water reabsorption in the distal tubule and early collecting ducts. They are not potent diuretics because only 5% of sodium reabsorption normally occurs at these sites. Thiazide diuretics are considered the first line of therapy for mild hypertension because of their diuretic effect. However, long-term benefits seem to come from vascular dilation and decreased peripheral vascular resistance.

24. Thiazide diuretics are considered the first line of therapy for mild _____ because of their diuretic effect.

## Potassium-sparing Diuretics

Potassium-sparing diuretics work in the distal tubule. Normally sodium is exchanged for potassium and hydrogen at this site to maintain an ion charge balance. Blocking sodium reabsorption at this site prevents potassium loss by secretion. Hyperkalemia can develop with use of these agents, so potassium levels should be monitored.

25. The most common diuretic combination is _____ and _____.

## ADVERSE EFFECTS

Although removal of fluid is the main goal of diuretic therapy, excessive fluid removal can lead to volume depletion or hypovolemia. Fluid load is a balance between input and output. Discontinuing a diuretic (decreasing output) should treat volume depletion caused by diuretics. If severe, IV fluid administration (increasing input) may be required.

Electrolyte imbalance is the second major complication with the use of diuretics. Hyperkalemia and hypokalemia are the two main concerns, with hyperkalemia being the more life-threatening of the two. It is difficult to predict which patients will develop an imbalance. Potassium supplementation is controversial but should be considered in patients with a history of heart disease or symptoms caused by low potassium, when serum potassium levels are less than 3.0 mEq/L, and for patients taking digitalis. The third complication is acid–base imbalance. Patients who have hypokalemia (and hypochloremia) may develop metabolic alkalosis as more hydrogen ion is secreted in exchange for potassium to maintain neutral fluid charges. Treatment with potassium and chloride should address this situation. Furosemide is one of the most effective and least toxic with pediatric patients. However, long-term use may cause nephrocalcinosis.

Increased blood glucose levels have been reported, especially with the use of loop and thiazide diuretics. Routinely these incidences have not been severe. The use of loop diuretics also has been associated with the development of ototoxicity, including tinnitus (ringing in the ears) and hearing loss, which are usually reversible. These side effects are related to drug blood level, so large doses and rapid infusions should be avoided.

26. List three major complications or adverse effects of diuretics:

a. _____

b. _____

c. _____

27. List three indications for potassium supplementation:

a. _____

b. _____

c. _____

28. An increased blood glucose level, called _____, is associated with the use of loop and thiazide diuretics.

29. One of the least toxic and most effective loop diuretics in pediatric practice is _____.

**206**

*The following represent five patients, each with a different problem. On the basis of the disease decide which of the five groups of diuretics to use. Use each diuretic group only once.*

30. Hypertension: _____

31. Edema, resistant to other drugs: _____

32. Glaucoma: _____

33. Head trauma: _____

34. Severe CHF with pulmonary edema: _____

## NATIONAL BOARD OF RESPIRATORY CARE–TYPE QUESTIONS

1. Which of the following statements is *not* true concerning diuretics?
   a. Diuretics increase urine output.
   b. Diuretics act directly on the kidney.
   c. Diuretics eliminate excess fluid from the body.
   d. Diuretics are all alike in their mode of action.

2. Carbonic anhydrase inhibitors act in which of the following?
   a. Proximal tubules
   b. Distal tubules
   c. Loop of Henle
   d. Glomerulus

3. Which of the following is *not* true concerning thiazide diuretics?
   a. They are potent diuretics.
   b. They act in the distal tubule.
   c. They are given orally.
   d. They may cause metabolic acidosis.

4. Potassium-sparing diuretics block which of the following?
   a. Potassium reabsorption
   b. Chloride reabsorption
   c. Bicarbonate reabsorption
   d. Sodium reabsorption

5. Normal urine output averages:
   a. 10–30 ml/hr
   b. 30–60 ml/hr
   c. 100–120 ml/hr
   d. 120–140 ml/hr

6. In a 70-kg person, how much of the total cardiac output flows through the kidney?
   a. 50%
   b. 40%
   c. 37%
   d. 22%

7. The functional unit of the kidneys is called a(n):
   a. Ureter
   b. Nephron
   c. Urethra
   d. Loop of Henle

8. Blood pressure and glomerular capillary blood flow influence the:
   a. Glomerular filtration rate
   b. Nephrons
   c. Blood flow from the heart
   d. Right heart pressure

9. In response to increased right heart pressure and stretch, _____ is released to increase urine output.
   a. Sodium
   b. Potassium
   c. Aldosterone
   d. Renin–angiotensin

10. If a patient has hypokalemia, which will force $Na^+$ exchange for $H^+$, the patient will develop:
    a. Respiratory acidosis
    b. Metabolic alkalosis
    c. Respiratory alkalosis
    d. Metabolic acidosis

11. The drug of choice to treat cerebral edema is:
    a. Furosemide
    b. Diamox
    c. Mannitol
    d. Benzthiazide

12. Patients receiving loop diuretics such as Lasix should have their _____ levels monitored.
    a. Bicarbonate
    b. pH
    c. Bleeding time
    d. Potassium

13. A patient receiving loop diuretics should experience diuresis within:
    a. 1 hour
    b. 20 minutes
    c. 2 hours
    d. 24 hours

14. The main reason for administering a loop diuretic to a patient with pulmonary edema is:
    a. To reduce inflammation in the airways
    b. To cause pulmonary artery vasoconstriction and reduce pulmonary vascular resistance
    c. To increase left heart pressure
    d. To cause diuresis and reduce pulmonary edema

15. For pediatric patients the least toxic and most effective loop diuretic is:
    a. Mannitol
    b. CAI
    c. Furosemide
    d. Isosorbide

Mrs. S has been brought to the emergency department with chief complaints of increasing shortness of breath, coughing, and mild substernal pressure. Her husband called the paramedics when Mrs. S complained that she "cannot breathe." She is currently on a nasal cannula at 4 L/min. Her husband states that she is a 66-year-old housewife with a history of coronary artery disease, arrhythmia, and a recent hospitalization for 3 weeks due to an anterior wall myocardial infarction (MI). She was discharged from the hospital 1 month ago after being treated for the anterior wall MI. Physical examination reveals her heart rate is 158 beats/min, her blood pressure is 110/70, and her $SpO_2$ (oxygen saturation by pulse oximetry) is 90%. Breath sounds have inspiratory crackles from the bases up to the midchest, with some expiratory wheezes. Her respiratory rate is 34 breaths/min with some paradoxical respirations noted. Pitting edema is present in the ankles, no clubbing or cyanosis is noted, and her skin is cool and diaphoretic. She has jugular vein distention.

1. On the basis of her physical findings in the emergency department, what immediate change in her care would you recommend?

She has been admitted to the cardiac care unit. A portable chest X-ray taken on admission in the emergency department has now been returned and reveals cardiomegaly, and bilateral pulmonary vascular engorgement with interstitial and alveolar edema. There is no pleural effusion or hemopneumothorax.

2. On the basis of her examination in the emergency room and her chest X-ray, what is her diagnosis?

3. What drug would be beneficial in helping to remove fluid from the patient's lungs?

4. Thirty minutes after giving 40 mg of Lasix, diuresis has not occurred. What would you now recommend?

It has been 2 hours since being admitted to the cardiac care unit. Mrs. S is resting more comfortably and she is on a nasal cannula at 3 L/min. Because of the medications she is currently receiving, chemistry laboratory tests are obtained with the following results:

Sodium: 140 mEq/L
Potassium: 2.6 mEq/L
Chloride: 87 mEq/L
Glucose: 125 mg/dl

5. On the basis of the chemistry results what would you recommend?

6. What acid–base imbalance could occur with these chemistry results?

7. What would you recommend for the treatment of the acid–base balance?

Chapter **21 Diuretic Agents**

# 22 Drugs Affecting the Central Nervous System

## CHAPTER OBJECTIVES

*After answering the following questions, the reader should be able to:*

1. Describe the multiple functions of the central nervous system.
2. Recognize various effects of medications on the central nervous system and their ability to modulate neurotransmitters.
3. Comprehend psychiatric medications, including their classification, use, and side effect profiles.
4. Recognize the effects of alcohol on the central nervous system during acute intoxication, chronic use, and after abrupt withdrawal.
5. Distinguish physiological and psychological bases of pain and the classes of analgesics used to treat them.
6. Recognize the indications for use of both local and general anesthesia.
7. Describe the concept of conscious sedation, and its indications and guidelines for use.
8. Distinguish drugs that stimulate the central nervous and respiratory systems and describe the indications for application.

## KEY TERMS AND DEFINITIONS

*Match the following definitions with their terms.*

1. _____ The brain and spinal cord make up the functional components of this system; together these provide for all conscious and subconscious functions of the body

2. _____ These drugs can alter levels of certain neurotransmitters, in particular norepinephrine and serotonin within the brain

3. _____ These drugs depress the nervous system. They can be divided into two categories, local and general

4. _____ These drugs are used primarily to treat bipolar disorders

5. _____ These drugs provide pain relief. They can be subdivided into narcotic and nonnarcotic medications

6. _____ These drugs are used to treat psychotic disorders, such as schizophrenia, and they affect primarily the neurotransmitter dopamine

7. _____ This is a method used during certain invasive procedures. The goal of this method is to decrease the level of consciousness, and relieve anxiety and pain, while allowing the patient to follow verbal commands

a. Analgesics
b. Anesthetics
c. Antidepressants
d. Antipsychotics
e. Anxiolytics
f. Central nervous system
g. Cholinesterase inhibitors
h. Conscious sedation
i. Mood stabilizers
j. Neurotransmitter
k. Stimulants

**211**

8. _____ These drugs can cause increased activity of the brain. They can be divided into two classes, the amphetamines and respiratory stimulants

9. _____ These drugs are known as minor tranquilizers. They treat several conditions, including anxiety disorders and insomnia

10. _____ These drugs block the activity of cholinesterase, an enzyme that inactivates the neurotransmitter acetylcholine

11. _____ This is a chemical substance that allows neurons to transmit electrical impulses throughout the central and peripheral nervous systems

## BRAIN STRUCTURE AND FUNCTION

The brain is made up of four main divisions: cerebrum, diencephalon, brainstem, and cerebellum. The cerebrum is the largest part of the brain. It is divided into two hemispheres and has several lobes. It is responsible for many functions, including but not limited to the five senses, motor and intellectual functions, memory storage, personality, behavior, and emotions.

The diencephalon contains the thalamus and hypothalamus. The thalamus is a relay station for most sensory fibers coming from the spinal cord to the cerebrum. The hypothalamus helps regulate body processes such as body temperature, water balance, and metabolism. It also controls pituitary gland function, which has a widespread effect on the body.

The brainstem has three parts: midbrain (mesencephalon), pons, and medulla. The brainstem relays information from the spinal cord to higher brain centers. The pons and medulla contain important centers for control of breathing.

The cerebellum sits at the posterior base of the skull. It is involved primarily with coordination of voluntary muscle activity.

The neuronal circuitry of the brain is enormously complex. Drugs that affect the central nervous system (CNS) will have widespread and varying effects.

12. Name three parts of the brain:

    a. _____

    b. _____

    c. _____

13. What disease is caused by a loss of neurons containing dopamine in the midbrain and is characterized by resting tremor and gait disturbances?

## NEUROTRANSMITTERS

The commonly considered neurotransmitters include norepinephrine, dopamine, and acetylcholine. The effect caused by any given neurotransmitter will vary depending on several factors, including but not limited to the amount released, the presence of transporting proteins, the efficiency of the reuptake process, and the presence of substances causing transmitter degradation. See Table 22-1 in the textbook for examples of neurotransmitters.

14. Name three common neurotransmitters.

    a. _____

    b. _____

    c. _____

## PSYCHIATRIC MEDICATIONS

Depression is a major cause of disability worldwide and one of the most common psychiatric disorders. It is likely caused by reduced activity of neurons in the limbic system. (The limbic system overlaps several areas in the brain and is involved with emotional states and behavior.) The drugs used to treat depression are listed in Tables 22-2 and 22-3 in the textbook. Side effects from the use of these drugs are multiple.

### Antidepressants

15. _____ and _____ have been shown to be important neurotransmitters, and their relative deficiency has been linked to depression.

### Mood Stabilizers
(*Hint:* See Table 22-4 in the textbook.)

16. Medical treatment of any pole of bipolar disorder must begin with a _____

    _____.

17. _____ disorder involves alternating episodes of depression and mania or hypomania.

### Antipsychotics

18. Pharmacotherapy for psychosis associated with depression or mania is generally used to increase

    _____ in the brain.

### Drugs for Alzheimer's Dementia

Alzheimer's dementia is associated with cognitive deficits secondary to decreased acetylcholine levels within the brain. These drugs are listed in Table 22-6 in the textbook.

   Some drugs used to treat anxiety and insomnia are listed in Table 22-7 in the textbook. Other drugs, used to induce sleep, are presented in Table 22-8 in the textbook.

19. What type of drug improves cognition and function in patients with Alzheimer's disease?

### Barbiturates and Other Hypnotics

Barbiturates are sedative agents that have been largely replaced by benzodiazepines because of potential toxic side effects, development of tolerance, and risk of addiction.

20. Given the following drug, give the indication for the drug.

a. Thiopental: _____

b. Pentobarbital: _____

c. Phenobarbital: _____

21. A common complaint that frequently results in the prescription of a hypnotic is _____

_____.

## ETHYL ALCOHOL

Alcohol is a by-product of sugar fermentation. It is used as a socially acceptable nonprescription, sedative-hypnotic agent. Ingested to excess, it behaves like a general anesthetic, depressing all brain areas, resulting in loss of voluntary muscle control and consciousness. At toxic levels (400 to 600 mg/dl, blood alcohol level) the respiratory center is affected and death as a result of respiratory arrest is likely.

22. Abrupt withdrawal after prolonged use may result in the syndrome of _____

_____, characterized by central nervous system hyperactivity, including hyperthermia, increased blood pressure, muscle twitching, hallucinosis, and seizures.

23. True or False: Alcohol is metabolized to $CO_2$ and $H_2O$, producing acetaldehyde in the process.

## PAIN TREATMENT

Pain is the subjective feeling that something hurts. Each of us handles pain in our own way and tolerates it to different degrees. Pain control is now an area of major concern in hospitalized patients. Analgesics (pain relievers) and nonanalgesic agents can affect perception and tolerance of pain. Inappropriate pain control can lead to unnecessary suffering and prolong patient recovery. Antidepressants combined with analgesics are used to treat chronic pain.

24. Nonanalgesic drugs such as barbiturates combined with _____ seem to decrease the experience of pain.

25. True or False: Chronic pain can be controlled by a combination of antidepressants and analgesics.

### Nonsteroidal Antiinflammatory Drugs

Nonsteroidal antiinflammatory drugs (NSAIDs) are used to treat moderate pain. They affect the hypothalamus and inhibit prostaglandin production. Aspirin and Tylenol are examples of NSAIDs. Aspirin causes gastric irritation, inhibits platelet aggregation, and is associated with the development of Reyes syndrome in adolescents and children. Tylenol is safer than aspirin in these regards.

### Opioid Analgesics

Opioid receptors exist in the brain and spinal cord. Endogenous (produced in the body) opioids, endorphins and enkephalins, modify pain perception. Narcotic (opioid) analgesics bind at these same receptors and are used to treat moderate to severe pain. High doses of opioids can lead to unconsciousness, respiratory arrest, and death. They have minimal effect on the cardiovascular system. Opioids produce a euphoric effect, but tolerance develops rapidly. Opioids are highly addictive, and drug withdrawal is an unpleasant experience. Morphine, codeine, heroin, and meperidine (Demerol) are common opioid receptor agonists. A few opioids are antagonistic at the mediator sites and can be used to reverse the analgesic and respiratory depression of the receptor agonists. Naloxone (Narcan) is one example of an opioid antagonist.

Opioids can be administered by several routes. IV administration via patient-controlled analgesia (PCA) devices is a common method for delivering opioids in a hospital setting. The oral route is another common method. Opioid delivery by inhalation is effective for pain control but is not widely used for medical purposes. See Table 22-10 in the textbook for a list of opioids.

## Local Anesthetics

Local anesthetics (Xylocaine, Novocaine) can be used to block pain nerve transmission from the damaged area. There is some evidence suggesting that systemic administration or inhalation may also enhance bronchodilation in asthma, as well as suppress irritant tracheal cough responses. Table 22-11 presents a list of local anesthetics.

## Epidural Analgesia

Both local anesthetics and opioids can be administered via continual epidural infusions. The epidural space surrounds the dura mater of the brain and spinal cord. Lumbar punctures are performed most commonly. Epidurals have a wide application in anesthesia because of their safety and versatility. Improved pain control has been achieved with the use of epidural catheters with minimal effect on normal sensory and motor function. Common uses include postoperative pain management and during labor and delivery.

26. The most frequently used analgesic, an NSAID that is purchased over the counter, is _____.

27. What would be a reason for suggesting aspirin over acetaminophen (Tylenol)?

28. If the Tylenol or aspirin doesn't take care of the pain, what would be the next agent you would suggest? Also, give an example of this agent.

29. One of the most serious side effects of opioids is respiratory depression. What drug could be used to reverse the respiratory depression?

30. True or False: Inhalation of local anesthetics may cause worsening bronchoconstriction as well as irritate the lungs, causing increased coughing.

## CHRONIC PAIN SYNDROMES

Chronic pain syndrome is believed to develop when peripheral pain leads to a central sensitization and presence of persistent pain even after the peripheral condition has resolved. The goal of pain therapy is to appropriately treat peripheral pain, while preventing central sensitization and chronic pain syndrome.

## ANESTHESIA

General anesthesia is a drug-induced state resulting in absence of perception. More than one drug group may be involved in achieving the desired goal of anesthesia and analgesia. Appropriate anesthesia is often determined by the patient's response to painful stimuli. The ideal anesthetic would include a pleasant and rapid induction and emergence, rapid changes of depth of anesthesia to match surgical demands, skeletal muscle relaxation to facilitate surgical exposure, a wide margin of safety, and no toxic or adverse effects. See Table 22-13 in the textbook for the more common anesthetic agents.

31. Depth of anesthesia is determined by patient response to painful stimuli and is often judged by the sympathetic

response, that is, a change in _____ _____ or

_____ _____.

## Conscious Sedation

Conscious sedation is light sedation that helps to eliminate a patient's pain and apprehension during clinical interventions. It allows patients to communicate and independently respond to appropriate verbal and physical stimuli. The inability to predict how patients will respond to light sedation requires close monitoring of these patients. As implied in the name, sedated patients should remain conscious and able to communicate, protect their own airway, and breathe adequately. Because most of the serious complications of conscious sedation relate to airway compromise, respiratory therapists are uniquely qualified to safeguard patients and improve outcomes during conscious sedation.

32. Several guidelines suggest that deep sedation and general anesthesia are indistinguishable. Because of this, how many qualified people must be continuously present during the sedation period?

33. Because of the potential for airway compromise, what should the respiratory therapist have available in order to maintain a patent airway?

34. According to Table 22-15 in the textbook, what recommendations for monitoring are suggested during conscious sedation?

   a. _____

   b. _____

   c. _____

   d. _____

## CNS AND RESPIRATORY STIMULANTS

Agents that stimulate brain activity are called analeptic drugs. Most of the stimulant drugs are sympathomimetics, acting directly on $\alpha$ and $\beta$ receptors. Their abuse potential is high and their side effects are predictable. They interfere with sleep and are used (and abused) to promote wakefulness and weight loss. Table 22-16 in the textbook contains a few common examples of CNS-stimulating drugs and their uses.

35. _____ is a common component in popular beverages and is used therapeutically in apnea–bradycardia syndromes of premature births.

36. True or False: Instead of using respiratory stimulants to treat elevated $Paco_2$ caused by muscle fatigue from increased work of breathing during mechanical ventilation, muscle rest and bronchodilation are more appropriate measures.

37. True or False: Respiratory stimulants have no clinical role in treating respiratory failure.

38. True or False: Methylxanthines, used to promote bronchodilation, also increase catecholamines and increase ventilation.

## NATIONAL BOARD OF RESPIRATORY CARE–TYPE QUESTIONS

1. The area of the brain that controls motor function and coordinates movement is the:
   a. Cerebrum
   b. Diencephalon
   c. Brainstem
   d. Cerebellum

2. Control of breathing is regulated mainly in the:
   a. Cerebrum
   b. Diencephalon
   c. Brainstem
   d. Cerebellum

3. For psychotic illnesses, drug therapy is directed at reducing the effects of which neurotransmitter?
   a. Norepinephrine
   b. Serotonin
   c. Dopamine
   d. Acetylcholine

4. Which of the following statements is *not* correct concerning alcohol?
   a. Withdrawal symptoms can be prevented by the use of sedative drugs.
   b. Chronic use results in the development of tolerance to its intoxicating effects.
   c. Malnutrition is seen with chronic use.
   d. When combined with other sedative drugs, the effect is synergistic.

5. Which of the following is correct concerning pain?
   a. It is an objective determination.
   b. Used alone, sedatives appear to increase perceived pain.
   c. Recall of pain intensity does not diminish with time.
   d. Both a and b

6. Which of the following is *not* a side effect of opioids?
   a. Diarrhea
   b. Constriction of pupils
   c. Respiratory depression
   d. Cough suppression

7. Which class of analgesics may enhance bronchodilation and suppress cough when administered via inhalation?
   a. Alcohol
   b. NSAIDs
   c. Local anesthetics
   d. Barbiturates

8. Depth of anesthesia is *best* determined by:
   a. Change in blood pressure
   b. ECG monitoring
   c. Response to painful stimuli
   d. Response to verbal commands

9. Which of the following are functional components of the central nervous system?
   I. Brain
   II. Spinal cord
   III. Heart
   IV. Lungs

a. I and II only
b. II and III only
c. I, II, and III only
d. II and IV only

10. Which of the following drugs are primarily used to treat bipolar disorders?
a. Stimulants
b. Antipsychotics
c. Mood stabilizers
d. Antidepressants

11. These drugs, subdivided into narcotic and nonnarcotic medications, provide pain relief:
a. Anxiolytics
b. Mood stabilizers
c. Analgesics
d. Cholinesterase inhibitors

12. Which of the following is *not* a part of the brain?
a. Pons
b. Spinal cord
c. Medulla
d. Midbrain

13. Which of the following is *not* a common neurotransmitter?
a. Catecholamine
b. Dopamine
c. Norepinephrine
d. Acetylcholine

14. Pharmacotherapy for psychosis associated with depression or mania is generally used to increase which of the following in the brain?
a. Norepinephrine
b. Dopamine
c. Acetylcholine
d. Catecholamine

15. A person diagnosed with Alzheimer's disease would have improvement of cognition and function with the use of this class of drugs:
a. Mood stabilizers
b. Sympathomimetics
c. Cholinesterase inhibitors
d. Pain relievers

16. Which of the following drugs is recommended to control seizures?
a. Thiopental
b. Pentobarbital
c. Norepinephrine
d. Phenobarbital

17. As alcohol is broken down and metabolized into $CO_2$ and $H_2O$, the by-product is:
a. Acetaldehyde
b. Dopamine
c. Norepinephrine
d. Acetylcysteine

18. Chronic pain can be controlled by antidepressants and _____.
a. Mood stabilizers
b. Analgesics
c. Tranquilizers
d. Anesthetics

19. The most frequently used analgesic NSAID that can be purchased over the counter is:
    a. Lithium
    b. Ethanol
    c. Aspirin
    d. Phenobarbital

20. Which of the following are opioid analgesics that produce a euphoric effect and are effective for pain relief?
    I. Morphine
    II. Codeine
    III. Demerol
    IV. Aspirin
       a. I and II only
       b. II and III only
       c. I, II, and III only
       d. II, III, and IV only

21. Which of the following are NSAIDs that are used to treat moderate pain and can be purchased over the counter?
    I. Aspirin
    II. Tylenol #3 with codeine
    III. Tylenol
    IV. Pentobarbital
       a. II and III only
       b. I and III only
       c. II and IV only
       d. I, II, and III only

22. Depth of anesthesia is determined by patient response to painful stimuli and is often judged by the sympathetic response, which is:
    a. Twitching of the extremities
    b. Lack of feeling in the extremities
    c. A change in heart rate or blood pressure
    d. A drop in arterial oxygen saturation

23. Because deep sedation and general anesthesia are indistinguishable, how many qualified people must be continuously present when administering conscious sedation?
    a. 2
    b. 3
    c. 4
    d. 5

24. The respiratory therapist is responsible for having _____ _____ available during conscious sedation in case there is a need to establish an emergency airway.
    a. Resuscitation equipment
    b. A mechanical ventilator
    c. A BiPAP ventilator
    d. A resuscitation bag

25. Respiratory failure resulting from sedative or opioid drug overdose can be treated with which of the following specific antagonists?
    a. Methylxanthines
    b. Morphine
    c. Naloxone
    d. Caffeine

You are the day-shift respiratory therapy supervisor and you will be involved in treating various patients throughout the day for different problems. Your travels today will take you to the emergency department (ED), the intensive care unit (ICU), labor and delivery, and neonatal ICU. Your task, if you decide to take it, will be to assist in decision-making opportunities in treating these patients. Good luck.

You are called to the ED, where you find that Mr. Jones, a 67-year-old COPD patient, has been admitted with pneumonia. His respiratory rate is 34 breaths/min, prolonged exhalation, accessory muscle usage and he is breathing with a 2-L/min nasal cannula. His ABG (arterial blood gas) shows the following: pH, 7.21; $Paco_2$, 74 mmHg; $Pao2$, 49 mmHg; $HCO_3$, 34 mEq/L. The resident wants to give a respiratory stimulant, an analeptic drug, to stimulate his breathing to "blow off" the $CO_2$. You enter the patient's room just as the resident is asking the nurse to give the drug.

1. What would you recommend?

You are now called to the adult ICU, where a patient is to receive conscious sedation before a procedure. As you enter the patient's room you look around and find no respiratory equipment.

2. Why should you obtain respiratory equipment to help in monitoring this patient during the procedure?

3. What should be continuously monitored and assessed during conscious sedation?

After leaving the adult ICU you are paged to labor and delivery, where a 32-week gestational age infant is born via cesarean section. The mother received several drugs, one of which was an opioid. The infant is not responding to typical stimuli and is currently being hand ventilated with a resuscitation bag.

4. What drug should be given to reverse the effects of the opioid?

From here you are called to neonatal ICU. The respiratory therapist is about to implement continuous positive airway pressure (CPAP) therapy on a 27-week infant who had been receiving mechanical ventilation. The therapist has reported to you that the infant has had some episodes of apnea and is concerned about placing the infant on CPAP. The therapist asks you to recommend a drug that would stimulate the infant's breathing.

5. What would you recommend?

# Answer Key

## CHAPTER 1

1. Drug
2. Pharmacology
3. Pharmacokinetics
4. Pharmacodynamics
5. *Pseudomonas aeruginosa*
6. Toxicology
7. Generic name
8. Respiratory syncytial virus
9. Chemical name
10. Therapeutics
11. Code
12. Trade
13. Chemical
14. Official
15. Generic
16.
    a. 4-(5-Cyclopentyloxy-carbonylamino-1-methyl-indol-3-ylmethyl)-3-methoxy-*N*-*o*-tolylsulfonylbenzamide
    b. ICI 204,219
    c. Zafirlukast
    d. Zafirlukast
    e. Accolate
17. United States Pharmacopeia–National Formulary (USP–NF)
18. The *Physician's Desk Reference*
19. The Hospital Formulary
20. Plants, minerals, animals
21. Antiasthmatic
22. Wizard of Oz
23.
    a. Phase 1: includes a small number of health subjects
    b. Phase 2: includes a small number of people who have the disease that the drug will treat
    c. Phase 3: includes a large number of people with the disease at different centers around the country
24. 6
25. AA
26. B
27. A
28. C
29. Advantage: It's good that there's a drug available to treat rare diseases.
30. Disadvantage: It's expensive to develop and market the drug.
31.
    a. Patient's name, address, date
    b. Rx, meaning recipe; this is the superscription
    c. Inscription, name of drug and the amount prescribed
    d. Subscription, direction to the pharmacist about preparation
    e. "Sig," directions to the patient (some medications must be taken on an empty stomach, some with milk; how many tablets, how many times a day, etc.)
    f. Prescriber's name, that is, the physician's name.
32. Primatene mist
33. True
34. There are five advantages of aerosolized agents given by inhalation. These include the following: a. Smaller doses may be given because the drug is acting directly on the airway; b. Side effects are usually fewer and less severe (partly because of the smaller dose); c. Onset of action is quick; d. Delivery of the drug is targeted to the respiratory system; e. Inhalation of aerosol drugs is painless, safe, and convenient.
35. Table of agents, effects of the agent, and example of the medication:

| Drug Group | Therapeutic Purpose | Agent |
|---|---|---|
| Adrenergic | Bronchodilation | Albuterol |
| Anticholinergic | Relaxation of bronchoconstriction | Atrovent |
| Mucoactive | Decrease in mucus viscosity | Mucomyst |
| Corticosteroid | Reduction of airway inflammation | Flovent |
| Antiasthmatic | Inhibition of chemical mediators | Intal |
| Antiinfective | Elimination of infective agents | Ribavirin |
| Surfactant | Increase in lung compliance | Infasurf |

36.
    a. Every 4 hours
    b. Every day
    c. Twice daily
    d. And
    e. Cubic centimeter
    f. A drop
    g. Intramuscular
    h. Liter
    i. Milliliter
    j. By mouth
    k. Every
    l. As needed
    m. A spray
    n. Nothing by mouth

o. Every hour
p. Every other day
q. Every 3 hours
r. Four times daily
s. Every 2 hours
t. Three times daily
u. Intravenous
37. Antiinfective drugs
38. Neuromuscular blocking agents
39. Analgesics
40. Antiarrhythmic
41. Antihypertensive and antianginal
42. Anticoagulants and thrombolytics
43. Diuretic
44. 1. c; 2. b; 3. g; 4. a; 5. f; 6. d; 7. e

**NBRC-type Questions**

1. d
2. b
3. b
4. c
5. a
6. b
7. a
8. d
9. c
10. c

**CHAPTER 2**

1. j
2. h
3. a
4. c
5. d
6. f
7. g
8. i
9. e
10. b
11. Drug dosage
12. Route of administration
13.
   a. Parenteral: tablet, capsule, suppository, elixir, suspension
   b. Enteral: solution, suspension, depot
   c. Inhalation: gas aerosol
   d. Transdermal: patch, paste
   e. Topical: powder, lotion, ointment, solution
14. Pharmacokinetic
15. Pharmacodynamic
16.
   a. Airway surface liquid
   b. Epithelial cells
   c. Basement membrane
   d. Interstitium
   e. Capillary vascular network
17. Aqueous
18. Lipid
19. Carrier-mediated

20. Pinocytosis
21. Bioavailability
22. Nonionized, lipid soluble
23.
   a. 5
   b. 10
   c. 20
   d. 14-25
24. $V_D \times$ concentration

$$100 \text{ mg} = V_D \times 5 \text{ mg/L}$$
$$V_D = 100/5 = 20 \text{ L}$$

25. Water
26. Liver
27. Abuse
28. Half-life
29. First-pass
30. Kidney
31. Clearance, plasma
32. Plasma half-life
33. True
34. True
35. Elimination
36. Drug A
37. Drug C
38. Drug B
39. *Local effect:* A drug affects the tissue with which it comes into direct contact. *Systemic effect:* A drug is absorbed and distributed in the blood stream
40. *Local:* Proventil, Ventolin. *Systemic:* Inhaled insulin
41. Lung and gastrointestinal
42. 90%
43. 10%
44. 50%-60%
45. Fewer systemic side effects
46. Reservoir device or holding chamber
47. True
48. Aerosol
49.
   a. Efficient delivery devices
   b. Inhaled drugs with high first-pass metabolism
   c. Mouthwashing, including rinsing and spitting
   d. Use of a reservoir device (spacer or holding chamber). All of the factors will increase delivery of aerosol into the lung and cause less drug to be swallowed.
50. False
51. Receptor
52. Fewer
53. Receptor proteins
54. G, adenylcyclase, transmembrane signaling
55. Concentration
56. Maximal effect
57. Drug B
58. Dangerous
59. Agonist
60. True
61. Less efficiency
62. Agonist

63. Antagonist
64. $1 + 1 = 2$
65. $1 + 1 = 3$
66.
    a. Potentiation
    b. Synergism
    c. Additivity
67. Potentiation
68. Idiosyncratic
69. Hypersensitivity
70. Tolerance
71. Tachyphylaxis
72. When a patient is challenged with a drug

## NBRC-type Questions

1. c
2. b
3. a
4. d
5. c
6. b
7. a
8. a
9. c
10. d
11. c
12. b
13. a
14. a
15. d
16. c
17. a
18. d
19. b
20. a

## Case Study

1. The oral and the parenteral routes are likely choices by which to give antibiotics. Because R.E.'s pneumonia seems to be advanced, the parenteral route (IV) will get the drugs into his system quicker than the oral route. R.E. will probably also receive a bronchodilator to treat his wheezing, with drug delivered via the inhalation route.
2. R.E. should receive a bronchodilator with a more complex chemical structure, so that it will only match with the $\beta_2$ receptors. This will give the patient bronchodilation without cardiac side effects. A good choice would be albuterol (with an intermediate time–plasma curve; refer to Figure 2-5).
3. 10%! He's right. He actually swallows most of the drug!
4. The spacer device will decrease oropharyngeal deposition and amount of drug swallowed.

## CHAPTER 3

1. Dead volume
2. In vitro
3. Aerodynamic diameter of a particle

4. CFC
5. Nebulizer
6. HFA
7. Reservoir device
8. Spacer
9. Deposition
10. Valved holding chamber
11. Penetration
12. Stability
13.
    a. To humidify inspired gas
    b. To improve the mobilization and elimination of secretions, such as a sputum induction (these aerosols can be water or saline)
    c. To deliver drugs to the respiratory tract
14. Advantages
    ■ Smaller doses can be used.
    ■ The drug acts quickly.
    ■ The drug goes right to the respiratory system.
    ■ There are fewer, less severe side effects (partly because smaller doses are used).
    ■ It's convenient and painless.
    Disadvantages
    ■ Many factors influence how much drug actually gets to the airways.
    ■ It's sometimes difficult to estimate the right dose; the same dose may not be delivered every time.
    ■ It's difficult for some people using an MDI to coordinate depressing the canister and inhaling. This is not as significant a problem now that there are spacers (reservoir devices).
    ■ The health care practitioner may not know all that he or she should about the device that the patient is using and/or how to use that device. (But whose fault is that?)
    ■ There is insufficient technical information about aerosol therapy devices.
15. 1-10 μm
16. 30, 50
17. Heterodisperse, polydisperse
18. True
19. Mass median aerodynamic diameter
20. Size
21. Nasal
22. 5-10 μm
23. 1-5 μm
24. 0.8-3.0 μm
25. The SVN delivering particles with an MMAD of 3.4 μm, because the particle size range required for lower airway delivery is 1-5 μm.
26. The SVN delivering particles with an MMAD of 7.9 μm, because the particle size range required to affect the upper airway is 5-10 μm.
27.
    a. Inertial impaction: Bigger particles, more turbulent flow, and higher velocities; these conditions favor inertial impaction on the airway wall, especially at airway bifurcations.

b. Gravitational settling: Bigger particles that move slower are more likely to fall out of suspension because of the force of gravity

c. Diffusion (Brownian motion): Particles less than 1 μm in size may either be exhaled or simply stay in suspension. (The time it takes for it to deposit anywhere is longer than a normal inspiration.)

28. Breathing
29. Slow, deep breaths with an inspiratory hold; through the mouth is best
30. Hygroscopic
31. USN is electrically powered, using the piezoelectric principle, and capable of high output. SVN is a gas-powered nebulizer with a small reservoir.
32.
   a. SVN
   b. Portable USN
   c. SVN
33. Covering the control port directs gas flow to the nebulizer, allowing nebulization to occur. Nebulization ceases when the hole is uncovered, because gas escapes through the uncovered hole.
34. The patient may be instructed to cover the hole when inhaling and to uncover it when exhaling.
35. Increasingly
36. True
37. True
38. False: Under clinical conditions of nebulization until sputter, approximately 35% to 60% of a drug solution is delivered from a nebulizer. Even with vigorous agitation, this amount increases to only 53% to 72%. Therefore the treatment is over at sputtering.
39. True
40. 3-5 ml
41. MMAD
42. 6 L/min, 10 L/min
43. Air or oxygen
44.
   a. 3-5 ml
   b. Approximately 5 minutes
   c. 6-10 L/min
   d. Air or oxygen
45. The dosimetric or breath-actuated SVN: Aerosol is released only during inspiration and all the released aerosol is available for patient inhalation.
46.
   a. Drug
   b. Propellant
   c. Canister
   d. Metering valve
   e. Mouthpiece/actuator
47. HFAs (hydrofluoroalkanes)
48. Hand–breathing
49. True
50. False: Shake the MDI before you use it to fill the metering valve and mix the suspension.
51. True
52. True
53. True
54. Corticosteroids
55.
   a. Increase drug delivery
   b. Reduced oropharyngeal deposition
   c. Improved coordination
56. Decrease, detergent. The effects of washing should last about 1 month.
57. A dry powder inhaler (DPI) is similar to a metered dose inhaler (MDI), that is, it is a small pressurized device for oral or nasal inhalation of aerosolized drugs, except that the drug is in powdered form and the device is breath-actuated.
58. 30-90 L/min
59. Exhale
60. True
61. True
62. False: There is no difference.
63. True
64. True
65. False: Two puffs of albuterol from an MDI contains 200 μg whereas an SVN of albuterol contains 2500 μg (0.5 cc, or 2.5 mg). If 10% of each is reaching the lung then the MDI administers 20 μg and the SVN administers 250 μg. It would take another 7–10 puffs to equal the dose provided by the SVN and to achieve the same clinical response. Remember that the amount of bronchodilation obtained is a reflection of the dose of drug given rather than the way it is delivered.
66.
   1. SVN, d
   2. MDI, a
   3. MDI with reservoir, c
   4. MDI with reservoir and mask, e
   5. MDI with ETT, b
   6. breath-actuated MDI, a
   7. DPI, a
67. SVN: volume of fill, type of solution, brand of SVN, intraproduct reliability, continuous versus intermittent, power flow rate. MDI: timing of actuation, use and design of reservoir device, type of drug used
68. Endotracheal tube
69. 30
70. Heat–moisture exchanger
71. Helium–oxygen mixture (also known as heliox)
72. 30%

**NBRC-type Questions**

1. c
2. a
3. d
4. a
5. d
6. b
7. d
8. c
9. d
10. a
11. a

12. c
13. a
14. c
15. d
16. a
17. b
18. d
19. b
20. c
21. d
22. c
23. b
24. c
25. b

**Case Study**

1. Based on the patient's information the most appropriate aerosol delivery device is an SVN.
2. Professor Plum has a high respiratory rate and because of this he is unable to breath-hold. The SVN is a simple method of administering aerosol medications and does not require him to focus on instructions. Just tell him to breath with the SVN. The SVN allows him to receive his medication over many breaths rather than trying to achieve the appropriate method of breathing that would be associated with an MDI. A DPI would be a bad choice for the same reasons, plus the professor may not be able to generate the necessary flow rate in the midst of his attack. When his respiratory rate begins to slow down the respiratory therapist can begin thinking about breath-holding for better deposition.
3. Now you can switch him to an MDI. (Remember, it's more cost-effective and easy to use.) His respiratory rate has now decreased, allowing him time to breath-hold. He is able to focus on instructions because he is no longer having severe breathing problems and he is now capable of performing the correct breathing maneuver for an MDI. This makes him a good candidate for an MDI.
4. He should use a reservoir device as this will increase the medication delivered to the lung. In addition, if his technique is not optimal, the reservoir device will help coordinate the aerosol delivery with his breathing. Not only will the reservoir increase the medication delivered, but if an antistatic device is chosen this will further increase the medication delivered. Otherwise you could instruct him to wash his regular reservoir with household detergent. It will reduce the electrostatic charge.

## CHAPTER 4

1. Strength
2. Percentage
3. Solution
4. Solute
5. Solvent
6. Schedule
7. 510

8. 33,000
9. 0.024
10. 1700
11. 68,000,000-68,000
12. 48
13. 8
14. 0.125

1 ml = 16 drops

$$\frac{1 \text{ ml}}{16 \text{ drops}} = \frac{x}{2 \text{ drops}}$$

$$\frac{16\,x}{x} = 2 \text{ drops}$$

$$= \frac{2}{16} \text{ or } 0.125 \text{ ml}$$

15. 2.5 tablets

Original dose = 200 mg (amount in 1 tablet)
Per amount = 1 tablet
Desired dose = 500 mg
Per amount = $x$ tablets

$$\frac{200 \text{ mg}}{1 \text{ tablet}} = \frac{500 \text{ mg}}{x \text{ tablets}}$$
$$500(1) = 200(x)$$
$$500 = 200(x)$$
$$x = 2.5 \text{ tablets}$$

16. 3 ml

Original dose = 10 mg
Per amount = 5 ml
Desired dose = 6 mg
Per amount = $x$ ml

$$\frac{10 \text{ mg}}{5 \text{ ml}} = \frac{6 \text{ mg}}{x \text{ ml}}$$
$$10(x) = 5(6)$$
$$x = \frac{30}{10} = 3 \text{ ml}$$

17. 0.000210 g
18. 0.50 ml

Original dose = 1 mg
Per amount = 1 ml
Desired dose = 0.5 mg
Per amount = $x$ ml

$$\frac{1 \text{ mg}}{1 \text{ ml}} = \frac{0.5 \text{ mg}}{x \text{ ml}}$$
$$1 \text{ mg}(x) = 0.50 \text{ mg}(1 \text{ ml})$$
$$x = 0.50 \text{ ml}$$

19. 4 ml/kg × 1.2 kg = 4.8 ml
20. 1 g/100 ml of solution: 0.001, which is 0.1% (0.001 × 100)
21. 10 mg
22. 20 mg

Percent strength = 1:250 = 0.004
Total amount of solution = 5 ml
Active ingredient = $x$
0.004 = $x$/5 ml
$x$ g = 0.004 × 5 = 0.02 g active ingredient, or 20 mg

23. 1.5 ml of 20% Mucomyst
    Percent strength (in decimals) = 0.10
    Total amount of solution = 3 ml
    Percent strength of solute = 0.20
    Dilute solute (active ingredient) = $x$ ml
    $0.10 = x(0.20)/3$ ml
    $x(0.20) = 0.10 \times 3$
    $x(0.20) = 0.30$
    $x = 0.3/0.20 = 1.5$ ml of 20% Mucomyst

24. They're the same. You're delivering 5 mg of drug in both cases; the only difference is that the treatment will take longer to administer with more diluent added.

## NBRC-type Questions

1. c
2. b
3. d
4. a
5. a
6. c
7. c
8. c
9. b
10. b

## Case Study 1

$$\text{Percent strength} = \frac{\text{solute (in grams or milliliters)}}{\text{total amount of solution}}$$

In this case first convert milligrams to grams: 20 mg = 0.02 g.

$$\text{Percent strength} = 0.02 \text{ g}/2 \text{ ml} = 0.01, \text{ or a}$$
$$1\% \text{ solution}$$

## Case Study 2

Percent strength (desired) = 0.20
Dilute solute (active ingredient) = $x$ ml
Percent strength of solute = 0.10
Total amount of solution = 6 ml
$0.20 = x(0.10)/6$ ml
$x(0.10) = 0.20 \times 6$
$x(0.10) = 1.2$
$x = 1.2/0.10 = 12$ ml of 10% Mucomyst.
(In general, this is mixed with some beverage to kill the yummy taste of Mucomyst.)

## CHAPTER 5

1. Central nervous system
2. Peripheral nervous system
3. Efferent
4. Afferent
5. Norepinephrine
6. Acetylcholine
7. Adrenergic
8. Anticholinergic
9. Parasympathomimetic
10. Sympatholytic
11. Parasympatholytic
12. Sympathomimetic
13. Nervous, endocrine
14.
   a. Central nervous system
   b. Peripheral nervous system
   c. Autonomic nervous system
15. Autonomic
16. Epinephrine
17. Craniosacral
18. Thoracolumbar
19.
   *Parasympathetic nervous system:*
   a. Essential to life
   b. Finely regulated
   c. Controls digestion, bladder, rectal function
   *Sympathetic nervous system:*
   a. General alarm system "fight or flight" response
   b. Not essential to life
   c. Increases heart rate and blood pressure, and blood flow shifts from periphery to core
20. Any life-threatening emergency requiring maximal physical exertion; if you've got to get out of a burning building, for example.
21. Nerve
22. Acetylcholine
23. Efferent. Remember that these impulses travel from the brain and spinal cord out to various sites (e.g., heart and lungs).
24. Acetylcholine
25. Cholinergic
26.
   1. e
   2. h
   3. g
   4. d
   5. c
   6. b
   7. f
   8. a
27.
   a. Slows rate
   b. Constriction
   c. Increased secretion
28. Nicotinic and muscarinic
29. Increase, because muscarine stimulates acetylcholine receptors in the exocrine glands (bronchial mucous glands).
30. Muscarinic, antimuscarinic
31. Methacholine (see Table 5-3 in the textbook).
32. Anticholinergic
33. Dramamine, because the anticholinergic effects are commonly used to prevent motion sickness.
34.
   a. Bronchodilation
   b. Treatment of bradycardia
   c. Preoperative drying of secretions
   d. Antidiarrheal agent. (More can be found in Box 5-1 in the textbook.)
35. Increase

36. Norepinephrine (except for sweat glands and the adrenal medulla)
37.
    a. Bronchodilator, cardiac stimulant, vasoconstrictor
    b. Bronchodilator
    c. Bronchodilator
    d. Antiarrhythmic
38. Alpha ($\alpha$) and beta ($\beta$)
39. Vasoconstriction
40. Rate, force of contraction
41. Bronchial, skeletal
42. $\alpha$ Receptors (vasoconstriction). If you dilated the vasculature of the nose the patient would be even more congested.
43. $\beta_2$ Receptors (relaxation of bronchial smooth muscle)
44. Sympatholytic
45. Epinephrine and norepinephrine
46. $\alpha$, $\beta$, $\alpha$
47. Relaxation
48. True
49. True
50. True
51. Pulmonary and bronchial
52. Parasympathetic nervous system, sympathetic nervous system
53. Sympathetic nervous system
54. Parasympathetic nervous system, sympathetic nervous system. When these glands are stimulated more mucus is produced.
55. $\alpha$, $\beta$
56. Vagus
57. Bronchoconstriction
58. Increase
59. $M_3$
60. Vasodilation (the relaxing factor that produces and is mediated by an increase in intracellular cGMP is nitric oxide)

## NBRC-type Questions

1. d
2. b
3. c
4. a
5. b
6. c
7. d
8. a
9. c
10. c
11. d
12. b
13. a
14. b
15. c
16. c
17. d
18. b
19. d
20. b

## Case Study 1

1. The parasympathetic effect is bronchoconstriction. Parasympathomimetic drugs such as methacholine are structurally similar to acetylcholine. They occupy cholinergic receptor sites at parasympathetic nerve terminals and cause activation of the receptor (bronchoconstriction). The more hyperreactive the airway, the greater the degree of bronchoconstriction in response to a certain dose of methacholine.
2. A methacholine challenge is useful in determining the degree of airway reactivity between asthmatic and nonasthmatic individuals and also in assessing the severity of that reactivity.

## CHAPTER 6

1. cGMP
2. Sympathomimetic
3. Bronchoconstriction
4. Catecholamines
5. Adrenergic bronchodilator
6. Prodrug
7. $\alpha$-Receptor stimulation
8. $\beta_1$-Receptor stimulation
9. Downregulation
10. $\beta_2$-Receptor stimulation
11. $\alpha$ Stimulation causes vasoconstriction and decongestion; $\beta_1$ stimulation causes increased heart rate and force of contraction.
12. Lung, heart
13. Relaxation of airway smooth muscle to reverse or lessen the degree of airflow obstruction
14. Albuterol, levalbuterol, perbuterol, terbutaline, metaproterenol, isoetharine, epinephrine
15. Asthma
16. Salmeterol, formoterol, and arformoterol
17. a. Bronchospasm; b. Nocturnal
18. Relievers, controllers
19. Dopamine, epinephrine, norepinephrine, isoproterenol, isoetharine
20. a, c, d, f
21. $\alpha$ and $\beta_1$ stimulation
22. Inhalation and subcutaneously
23. They are inactivated in the gut and liver.
24. No, because the medication needs to rain out in the upper airway.
25. a, b, and d
26. Mouth, MDI, aerosol, syrup
27. Effective by mouth, duration up to 6 hours, peak effect in 30–60 minutes, $\beta_2$-preferential effect
28. a, b, c, d
29. When it is given, it changes to something else in the body—and this becomes the active drug.
30. 8 hours
31. 0.31, 0.63, and 1.25 mg/3 ml; there is also a 1.25 mg/0.5 ml unit dose that can be used when adding another drug to this unit dose
32. HFA-propelled MDI
33. a, b, c

34.
   a. Arformoterol
   b. Salmeterol and formoterol
   c. Salmeterol, formoterol, and arformoterol
   d. Salmeterol
   e. Salmeterol, formoterol, and arformoterol
   f. Formoterol and arformoterol
35. 12 hours
36. $\beta_2$-Selective, dry powder
37. Salmeterol is a maintenance drug. Maintenance drugs would be of little or no benefit to a person having an asthma attack because these drugs are slow to peak.
38. 3 to 5, 12
39. Adults, children older than 5 years of age
40. Adults, children older than 12 years of age
41. 12, 2 to 3
42. Antiinflammatory
43.
   a. T
   b. T
   c. F (short-acting agents are recommended because of their quick onset of action)
   d. T
   e. F
   f. T
   g. T
44. 12
45.
   a. 1
   b. 3
   c. 3
   d. 2
   e. 1
   f. 2
   g. 3
46.
   a. Y
   b. Y
   c. Y
   d. Y
   e. Y
   f. Y
   g. N
47. Rapid onset, smaller doses compared with oral route, reduced side effects, drug is delivered to target organ (lung), painless and safe
48. Catecholamines
49. Continuous nebulization
50. Ease, simplicity, short time required for administration (1 or 2 oral tablets vs. 4 inhalation treatments), exact reproducibility, and control of dosage
51. Any effect other than the intended therapeutic effect
52. Reduced effectiveness of a drug with use over time
53. Airflow changes; histamine, methacholine, cold air
54. Ventilation–perfusion
55.
   a. T
   b. T
   c. T

   d. F (antiinflammatory agents should also be emphasized, especially with patients who respond poorly to $\beta$ agonists); e. T; f. T

## NBRC-type Questions

1. a
2. b
3. d
4. c
5. b
6. d
7. b
8. d
9. d
10. d
11. c
12. b
13. a
14. d
15. a
16. c
17. b
18. d
19. a
20. d
21. b
22. b
23. a
24. c
25. c
26. a
27. c
28. c
29. b
30. d
31. b
32. c
33. a
34. d
35. d
36. c
37. d
38. a
39. c
40. a
41. b
42. d
43. c
44. d

## Case Study

1. Salmeterol would be an excellent choice to accompany the prophylactic and antiinflammatory agents because of its long-acting properties. Patients are much more likely to comply with therapy the less often a drug must be taken. This patient is already taking both cromolyn sodium and a corticosteroid. Why prescribe a bronchodilator that must be taken four times a day when a twice-daily choice is available? Because salmeterol lasts up to 12 hours it

is also a good choice, as it can control asthma overnight.

2. If this youngster has an asthma attack, salmeterol is not the adrenergic bronchodilator of choice! Remember, it doesn't peak for 3 to 5 hours, so it won't give him any relief during an asthma attack. And if he feels no relief, he may take another hit off the MDI—and another—until he experiences tachyphylaxis and cardiac side effects, which may result in death.

## CHAPTER 7

1. Parasympatholytic
2. Cholinergic
3. Anticholinergic bronchodilator
4. Muscarinic
5. Antimuscarinic
6. Parasympathomimetic
7.
    a. Ipratropium bromide
    b. Tiotropium bromide
8. Anticholinergic and β agonist
9. Ipratropium bromide and albuterol
10. Ipratropium bromide
11.
    a. Spiriva
    b. Atrovent
    c. Combivent
12.
    1. a and b
    2. a
    3. a
    4. a, b, and c
    5. c
13.

| | Adult Dosage | Time Course |
|---|---|---|
| Atrovent MDI | 18 μg/puff, 2 puffs qid | Onset: 15 min Peak: 1-2 hr Duration: 4-6 hr |
| Atrovent HFA MDI | 17 μg/puff, 2 puffs qid | Onset: 15 min Peak: 1-2 hr Duration: 4-6 hr |
| Combivent | MDI: Ipratropium 18 μg/puff and albuterol 90 μg/puff, 2 puffs qid | Onset: 15 min Peak: 1-2 hr Duration: 4-6 hr |
| DuoNeb | SVN: ipratropium 0.5 mg and albuterol 3.0 mg (equal to 2.5 mg albuterol base) | Onset: 15 min Peak: 1-2 hr Duration: 4-6 hr |
| Spiriva | DPI: 18 μg/ inhalation, 1 inhalation daily (1 capsule) | Onset: 30 min Peak: 3 hr Duration: 24 hr |

14. Atropine sulfate
15. Tertiary ammonium compound
16. Quaternary ammonium compound
17. Because tertiary ammonium compounds have greater side effects, quaternary ammonium compounds, such as Atrovent, are better choices for bronchodilation in the parasympatholytic class.
18.

| | Cholinergic Effect | Anticholinergic Effect |
|---|---|---|
| Decreased heart rate | X | |
| Drying of upper airway | | X |
| Salivation | X | |
| Mucociliary drying | | X |
| Secretion of mucus | X | |
| Bronchoconstriction | X | |
| Inhibition of bronchial constriction | | X |
| Increased heart rate | | X |

19.

| | Tertiary (e.g., Atropine) | Quaternary (e.g., Ipratropium) |
|---|---|---|
| Bronchodilation | X | X |
| Blocks hypersecretion | X | |
| No change in mucociliary clearance | | X |
| Slowing of heart rate with small dosage, increased heart rate with large dosage | | X |
| No heart rate effect | X | |
| Blocks nasal hypersecretion | | X |
| Decreased mucociliary clearance | X | |

20. Parasympathomimetic agent
21. Dry mouth, cough
22. True
23. True
24. True
25. False: It is not recommended, but if a facemask is used the eyes should be covered to prevent drug exposure. This is especially true for COPD patients, among whom narrow-angle glaucoma is more common.

26.

| | Anticholinergic | β Agonist |
|---|---|---|
| Onset | Slightly lower | Faster |
| Time to peak effect | Slower | Faster |
| Duration | Longer | Shorter |
| Fall in $Pa_{O_2}$ | None | Yes |
| Site of action | Larger, central airways | Central and peripheral airways |

27. COPD
28. Nocturnal asthma
29. β Agonists
30. Central, peripheral
31. True
32. $FEV_1$
33. Combivent and DuoNeb
34. False: It requires assessing pulse before, during, and after treatment.
35. True
36. False: The patient should be instructed in the use of all devices.
37. True

**NBRC-type Questions**

1. b
2. a
3. c
4. b
5. d
6. c
7. a
8. c
9. d
10. d
11. c
12. d
13. d
14. c
15. d

**Case Study**

Hopefully, you didn't pick either one. Trick question! The best choice for Jane is a combination of albuterol and ipratropium, for the following reasons:

| Anticholinergic | β Adrenergic |
|---|---|
| Acts on central airways | Acts on smaller airways |
| Peaks more slowly | Peaks sooner |
| Lasts longer | Terminates sooner |

All these effects are complementary, for the longest lasting relief. However, if you were forced to choose between sympathomimetic bronchodilators or anticholinergic bronchodilators, choose the anticholinergic agents. These have been proven to have at least some impact on improving airflow. Some patients with COPD may suffer bothersome side effects as a result of adrenergic bronchodilators anyway, because many of these patients have heart difficulties.

**CHAPTER 8**

1. Methylxanthines
2. Potential toxicity
3. It stimulates breathing
4. Caffeine citrate has a higher therapeutic index and fewer side effects compared with theophylline.
5.
   a. Caffeine
   b. Theophylline
   c. Theobromine
6.
   a. Sustained-release oral form
   b. As aminophylline for oral or intravenous administration
   c. Rectal suppository form
7.

| Effect | Caffeine | Theophylline |
|---|---|---|
| CNS stimulation | +++ | ++ |
| Smooth muscle relaxation | + | +++ |
| Skeletal muscle stimulation | +++ | ++ |
| Cardiac stimulation | + | +++ |
| Diuresis | + | +++ |

8.
   *Treatment of Asthma*
   a. 2
   b. 1
   c. 3.
   *Treatment of COPD*
   a. 2
   b. 1
   c. 3
9.

| Micrograms ($\mu$g)/milliliter (ml) | Effect |
|---|---|
| a. <5 | None |
| b. 10 to 20 | Therapeutic range |
| c. >20 | Nausea |
| d. >30 | Cardiac dysrhythmias |
| e. 40 to 45 | Seizures |

10. 5 to 15, 10 to 12
11. There is no therapeutic effect
12. Increase the dose
13. Decrease the dosage and determine a blood level
14. 1, 2
15. 5, 9

16.
 1. e
 2. c
 3. b
 4. a
 5. d
 6. b
 7. a
17. Because of the diuretic effect of theophylline, ensure that patients with excess airway secretions (e.g., those with bronchitis or cystic fibrosis) receive adequate fluid replacement to prevent dehydration and thickening of secretions.
18. Liver, kidney
19. True
20. True
21. True
22. False: Intravenous aminophylline is listed in the GOLD guidelines as one of several bronchoactive agents for the management of an acute exacerbation of COPD.
23. True
24. False: Theophylline can increase cardiac output, decrease pulmonary vascular resistance, and improve myocardial muscle perfusion in ischemic regions.
25. False: Caffeine is a more potent stimulator. It also has a wider therapeutic margin with fewer side effects.
26. True

**NBRC-type Questions**

 1. c
 2. b
 3. a
 4. b
 5. b
 6. d
 7. c
 8. a

15.

 9. a
10. d
11. c
12. d
13. d
14. c
15. c
16. c
17. d
18. a
19. c

**Case Study**

1. For long-term therapy, use 16 mg/kg/24 hr or 400 mg/24 hr, whichever is less. Joe's calculated dose is $16 \times 75 = 1200$ mg; 400 mg is less. So give him 400 mg the first day, which is 200 mg bid.
2. 5 to 9 hours after the morning dose
3. Because Joe's clinical presentation is unchanged and his level is low (the desired level is 10 to 12 μg/ml), his dose should be increased. Obtain another serum level and monitor him closely.

**CHAPTER 9**

 1. c
 2. f
 3. k
 4. b
 5. d
 6. m
 7. g
 8. j
 9. e
10. l
11. h
12. a
13. i
14. Mucoactive

| Drug | Brand Name | Use | Adult Dose |
|---|---|---|---|
| *N*-Acetylcysteine 10% | Mucomyst | Bronchitis (no clinical evidence to support its use) | SVN: 3-5 ml |
| Dornase alfa | Pulmozyme | CF | SVN: 2.5 mg/ampoule. One ampoule/day |
| Aqueous aerosols: water, saline | Not applicable | Sputum induction, secretion, mobilization | SVN: 3-5 ml |

16. False: There is no scientific evidence to support this finding.

17.

| Drug Group | Ciliary Beat | Mucus Production |
|---|---|---|
| β Adrenergic agents | Increase | Increase |
| Cholinergic agents | Increase | Increase |
| Methylxanthines | Increase | Increase |
| Corticosteroid | No effect | Decrease |

18. True
19. Tobacco smoke
20. True
21. *Pseudomonas*
22. Mucin, pus
23. Increase viscosity and mucus transport is impeded
24.
   a. When possible remove causative factors such as pollution and smoking, and treat infections
   b. Optimize tracheobronchial clearance including the use of bronchodilators and the incorporation of bronchial hygiene measures. These include coughing, deep breathing, postural drainage, and other airway clearance measures.
25. Disulfide bonds
26. Rapid-onset
27. False: This indicates metal ion removal and does not affect the efficacy of the drug. Opened vials should be discarded after 96 hours.
28. True
29. These secretions have a higher level of mucin and related proteins whereas CF secretions are almost entirely neutrophil-derived pus
30.
   a. Management of CF
   b. Reduction of the frequency of respiratory infections
   c. Preservation of lung function in patients with respiratory infections
31.
   a. Hudson Updraft II;
   b. Acorn II (both a and b use the DeVilbiss Pulmo-Aide compressor)
   c. Pari LC Jet Plus with Pari Inhaler Boy compressor
32. The drug is expensive; therefore optimal delivery of particle size and quantity is desirable.
33. There are several ways: 1. Reduction in IV antibiotic use; 2. Reduced need for hospitalizations; 3. Stability of lung function; 4. Reduced number and severity of infectious exacerbations
34. Asthma
35. CF and chronic bronchitis
36. Chronic bronchitis
37. CF
38. Ultrasonic nebulizer
39. True
40. True

41. False: The active cycle of breathing technique is a combination of breathing control (relaxed diaphragmatic breathing), thoracic expansion control (deep breaths), and forced expiration technique from progressively increasing lung volumes.
42. True
43. False: Exercise should be included with other bronchial hygiene regimens.
44. True
45. True
46. Flutter mucus clearance device
47. Intermittent percussive ventilation (IPV)
48. Chest wall oscillations: The Vest

**NBRC-type Questions**

1. a
2. c
3. d
4. a
5. d
6. c
7. c
8. b
9. d
10. b
11. a
12. d
13. a
14. a
15. c
16. b
17. d
18. c
19. d

**Additional Practice**

1. g
2. c
3. d
4. a
5. b
6. a
7. f
8. e

**Case Study**

1. He can use any of the following equipment: a Hudson Updraft II or Acorn II (both use a Pulmo-Aide compressor), or a Pari LC Jet Plus with Pari Inhaler Boy compressor. He should receive one 2.5-mg dornase alfa ampoule per day. His albuterol should be administered four times per day and along with his airway clearance with The Vest.
2. It is better to wait until Johnny is older than 8 years of age for autogenic drainage. It requires more concentration than other airway clearance techniques. And yes, the parents will be taught percussion and postural drainage.

3. The most common side effects for Pulmozyme are voice alteration, inflammation of the upper airway, chest pain, rash, and eye inflammation. Albuterol is a very safe drug. Johnny's pulse should be taken before, during, and after therapy.
4. No, he can sit in a chair while he is taking his nebulizers.
5. He should use it for 20–30 minutes; if he takes his nebulized medications at the same time this will save him some time.
6. The best airway clearance device is the one he is going to use each day. He may need to try several different types of airway clearance devices before he feels comfortable with one. Because you will know how to do percussion and postural drainage you can do that if he gets tired of The Vest. Since Johnny will be back in 2 weeks for a follow-up visit we'll meet again and evaluate his respiratory care.

## CHAPTER 10

1. Surfactant
2. Surface tension
3.
   a. The internal pressure of a drop or bubble
   b. The amount of surface tension
   c. The radius of the drop or bubble
4. Because there is only a single air–liquid interface.
5. Higher, collapse
6.

| Drug | Brand Name | Amount in Vial | Initial Dose |
|------|-----------|----------------|--------------|
| Beractant | Survanta | 8 ml | 4 ml/kg in four divided doses |
| Calfactant | Infasurf | 6 ml | 3 ml/kg in two divided doses of 1.5 ml/kg |
| Poractant alfa | Curosurf | 1.5-ml vial (120 mg of phospholipid) or 3-ml vial (240 mg of phospholipid) | 2.5 ml/kg in two divided doses |

7. RDS = respiratory distress syndrome
8. Prophylactic
9. High
10. To regulate surface tension forces of the liquid lining of the alveolus
11. Lecithin
12. Lamellar bodies
13. Surface tension, compliance
14. Increased volume with the same pressure change (see Figure 10-2 in the textbook)
15. Natural
16. Bovine, porcine

17.
   a. Prophylactic therapy of premature infants weighing less than 1250 g at birth or with evidence of surfactant deficiency and risk of RDS. Give the agent within 15 minutes of birth or as soon as possible.
   b. Rescue treatment of infants with evidence of RDS; the agent should be given within 8 hours of birth.
18. The recommended dose of beractant (Survanta) is 100 mg of phospholipids per kilogram of birth weight. Because there are 25 mg of phospholipids per milliliter in the beractant suspension, this is equivalent to a dose of 4 ml/kg of birth weight, in four divided doses.
19. False: The vial can be swirled but not shaken.
20. True
21. True
22. False: The infant is manually ventilated for 30 seconds between doses.
23.
   a. Prophylactic therapy of premature infants less than 29 weeks of gestational age and at risk of RDS
   b. Rescue treatment of premature infants less than or equal to 72 hours of age who develop RDS and require endotracheal intubation
24. 800 g = 0.80 kg, therefore $0.80 \times 3$ ml = 2.4 ml
25. True
26. True
27. Side-port administration: The patient should be positioned with either right or left side dependent with each aliquot delivery. Assess the patient before the second aliquot is delivered. Catheter administration: The dose is divided into four equal doses to be delivered in a different position (prone, supine, right lateral, and left lateral).
28.
   a. Rescue treatment of premature infants with RDS, reducing mortality and pneumothoraces
   b. Unlabeled uses: severe meconium aspiration syndrome (MAS) in term infants; respiratory failure caused by group B streptococcal (GBS) infection in neonates
29. $0.80$ kg $\times 2.5$ ml/kg = 2 ml
30. True
31. False: The vial should be turned upside down to uniformly disperse the suspension.
32. True
33. True: Otherwise no suctioning should occur for 1 hour.
34. True
35. The infant is positioned with either the right or left side down for the first aliquot. The infant is then changed to the opposite side for the second aliquot.
36.
   a. Improvement of oxygenation as seen by increased $PaO_2$, $SpO_2$ (oxygen saturation as determined by pulse oximetry), stable heart rate

b. Improved lung compliance as seen by better chest expansion, increased volume, less flattening of the pressure–volume curve (see Figure 10-1);

c. Increased functional residual capacity (FRC) as seen by less consolidation on chest radiograph.

## NBRC-type Questions

1. b
2. b
3. b
4. a
5. d
6. b
7. d
8. b
9. a
10. c
11. d
12. c
13. b
14. d
15. b
16. b
17. c
18. d
19. b
20. a
21. a

## Case Study

1. Present the following information:
   a. The baby's lungs are immature and have not yet manufactured enough surfactant to keep the lungs open to help the infant breathe.
   b. Surfactant makes it easier for oxygen to enter the air sacs because the surfactant allows the air sacs to remain open.
   c. The baby is working too hard to breathe. He will tire and require a longer stay on mechanical ventilation until his lungs mature sufficiently.
   d. The Survanta is artificial surfactant that can be given into the lungs. This will allow easier breathing.
   e. Once the baby gets the recommended dose, the surfactant will be recycled by his alveoli, and he has a greater chance of coming off the ventilator sooner. His chance of survival is likely to be better also.
2. Present the following information:
   a. He will have better oxygenation in the blood as seen by an increase in $SpO_2$, $PaO_2$, and heart rate.
   b. His breathing will improve.
   c. His respiratory rate will decrease and his work to breathe will become easier.
   d. As improvement continues we will start decreasing the parameters on the ventilator, such as the pressure and volume.
3. 20 minutes
4. The vial can be swirled gently but should not be shaken.

5. $0.90 \text{ kg} \times 3 = 2.7$ ml. Each aliquot is 1.35 ml.
6.
   a. Place the baby either right or left side dependent
   b. Give 1.35 ml through the side-port adaptor timed to coincide with inspiration
   c. Ventilate for 30 seconds
   d. Turn the baby to the opposite side in the dependent position
   e. Repeat the same procedure as for the first dose
   f. Ventilate for 30 seconds.
7. The baby can receive a total of three doses. The repeat doses can be given 12 hours apart.

## CHAPTER 11

1. Steroid diabetes
2. Endogenous
3. IgE
4. Prostaglandin
5. Steroids
6. Adrenal cortical hormones
7. Exogenous
8. Chemical mediators
9. a. Oral; b. Intranasal
10. Step 2 or greater
11. Systemic
12.
   a. Seasonal and perennial allergic rhinitis
   b. nonallergic rhinitis
13.
   a. 4
   b. 3
   c. 2
   d. 5
   e. 1
   f. 6
14.
   a. 6
   b. 2
   c. 5
   d. 4
   e. 3
   f. 1
15.
   a. Muscle wasting
   b. Steroid diabetes
16. Adrenal
17. Aerosolized
18.
   a. Asthma
   b. Chronic bronchitis
19.
   a. Redness: local dilation of blood vessels
   b. Flare: reddish color extending several centimeters from the site, occurring within 15-30 seconds
   c. Wheal: local swelling occurring within minutes
20. IgE
21.
   a. Decreased mucus secretion
   b. Decreased plasma leakage
   c. Restored responsiveness to β agonists

22. DPIs and HFA-propelled MDIs
23. 50, 60%
24. Spacer
25. Absorption
26. MDI, DPI
27. Pulmicort Respules can be mixed with other agents such as bronchodilators.
28. Fluticasone and salmeterol
29. Budesonide and formoterol
30. White blood cell
31. To restore β-adrenergic responsiveness
32. Bacterial, viral, and fungal
33. Adrenal insufficiency
34.
    a. Oropharyngeal candidiasis (oral thrush)
    b. Dysphonia
35.
    a. Mouth rinsing after administration (to clean out the oropharynx)
    b. Use of a spacer to decrease the amount of drug deposited at the back of the throat
    c. Giving the lowest dose possible
36. True
37. False: The shift was from the second line of defense to the first line of defense.
38. True
39. False: Mild, moderate, and severe persistent asthma can all be treated.
40. True
41. False: Cromolyn sodium, nedocromil sodium, and leukotriene modifiers are the initial choice for long-term control therapy of mild persistent asthma in children, because these medications have excellent safety profiles
42. Reduce systemic side effects, decrease amount of drug deposited in the oropharynx
43. A β₂ agonist can improve lung function.
44. Peak flow meter
45. Asthma is predominated by eosinophils, and COPD is predominated by neutrophils.
46. True

**NBRC-type Questions**
1. b
2. a
3. c
4. c
5. b
6. c
7. b
8. c
9. d
10. d
11. c
12. b
13. d
14. a
15. b
16. d
17. b

18. d
19. d

**Case Study 1**
**Asthma**
1. 100 μg/puff × 2 = 200 μg/treatment × 4 = 800 μg/day
2.
    a. Make sure that Mrs. Peacock can demonstrate proper MDI technique. (If you forget what this is, review CHAPTER 3.)
    b. Stress the importance of using a spacer device so that less of the drug is deposited in the back of her throat, so she's less likely to get a fungal infection.
    c. Tell her she will need to rinse her mouth and/or gargle after each treatment, as this will also minimize the chance of fungal infection.
    d. Let her know that she may also experience dysphonia (hoarseness or change in voice quality), cough, or mild bronchospasm, and that if she does, she should notify you to contact her physician and discuss other options. These would include other corticosteroids or a lower dose of triamcinolone.

**Case Study 2**
**Asthma**
1. Betty should be moved up to step 2 care. She could be given an inhaled antiinflammatory low-dose corticosteroid such as beclomethasone dipropionate or budesonide.
2. Betty needs to increase her inhaled corticosteroid dose to a medium dose, and she needs a long-acting bronchodilator especially for the night-time symptoms. A combination drug such as fluticasone/salmeterol would help Betty. Other drugs that could be added include sustained-release theophylline or long-acting β₂-agonist tablets.

**Case Study 3**
**COPD**
1.
    a. Oxygen by nasal cannula to raise the SpO₂
    b. Short-acting β₂ adrenergic and short-acting anticholinergic by SVN such as albuterol and ipratropium bromide
    c. IV glucocorticoids
    d. Empiric antibiotic therapy
2.
    a. Increased dyspnea (patient states he had increased shortness of breath)
    b. Increased sputum production
    c. Purulent-appearing sputum
3.
    a. *Haemophilus influenzae*
    b. *Streptococcus pneumoniae*

4. In Andy's case he had an infection, which is one of the most common reasons for exacerbation. The other reason is air pollution.
5.
   a. Combination short-acting $\beta_2$ agonist plus anticholinergic drug, such as albuterol and ipratropium bromide
   b. Combination long-acting $\beta_2$ agonist plus glucocorticoid, such as formoterol and budesonide.
6.
   a. Inhaled respiratory medications are required no more than four times daily;
   b. Andy has been clinically stable for 12-24 hours
   c. Andy fully understands the correct use of the respiratory medications he is to use at home, including the spacer device.

## CHAPTER 12

1. Mast cells
2. Mast cell stabilizers
3. Leukotrienes
4. Antileukotriene
5. Cromolyn-like drugs and antileukotrienes (anti-LTs)
6. Cromolyn sodium, nedocromil sodium
7. Controllers
8. The patient using a rescue $\beta_2$ agonist more than two times per week (i.e., in step 2 asthma)
9.
   a. R
   b. C
   c. C
   d. C
   e. C
   f. R
10.
   a. The acute asthma attack, which resolves spontaneously or with treatment
   b. Hyperresponsiveness of the airways to various stimuli
   c. Persistent inflammation that is now appreciated or becomes worse
11. Intal
12. 20
13. 2
14.
   a. Antiasthmatic
   b. Antiallergic
   c. Mast cell stabilizer
15. 2, 4
16. True
17. Controller, bronchodilator, acute
18. $8 \times 1.75$ mg = 14 mg
19.
   a. Zileuton (Zyflo)
   b. Montelukast (Singulair)
   c. Zafirlukast (Accolate)
20. Prophylaxis and chronic treatment of asthma
21. 12

22. One 600-mg tablet qid
23. Meals and bedtime
24. Hepatic transaminase enzymes
25. Theophylline and warfarin
26. 5
27. Exercise, allergen
28. 10, 20
29. 1, 2
30. 5
31. Tablet, granule
32. Liver
33. Steroids and antileukotrienes
34. Omalizumab reduces the mediators that can be released in an allergic reaction by blocking the binding of IgE to the IgE receptor on the surface of mast cells and basophils.
35. True
36. True
37. False: Xolair may reduce the need for rescue agents.

**NBRC-type Questions**

1. b
2. a
3. c
4. c
5. a
6. c
7. b
8. a
9. c
10. d
11. a
12. b
13. b
14. a
15. c

**Case Study**

1. Try cromolyn sodium first. It has been proven to be effective in EIB. Nedocromil sodium can also be recommended, but it has a bad taste—something Bruce may not want to experience as he is crossing the finish line.
2. Bruce can understand and follow directions, and can perform a slow inspiration with an inspiratory hold, so nothing precludes him from using an MDI. Therefore the delivery device of choice for Bruce is an MDI. It is the most easily carried device even though it provides a lower dose compared with a nebulized solution.
3. Bruce should take 2 puffs (2 mg/dose), 15 minutes before exercising. The total number of puffs is 2 puffs, 4 times a day.
4. Do not say that he should go home and get his cromolyn sodium MDI! Remember, bronchospasm should never be treated with an antiasthmatic. The purpose of an antiasthmatic is to prevent inflammation. Once the inflammation and bronchospasm have occurred, a $\beta$ agonist is needed.

He should have a fast-acting $\beta_2$ bronchodilator with him just in case of such a situation. Caution Mr. Jenkins that he should never exercise without taking his medications wherever he goes.

## CHAPTER 13

1. Virostatic
2. Respiratory syncytial virus
3. Cystic fibrosis
4. *Pneumocystis* pneumonia (PCP)
5. Virucidal
6. Virus
7.
   a. Prophylaxis for PCP, NebuPent
   b. Treatment of respiratory syncytial virus, Virazole
   c. For control of chronic *P. aeruginosa* infection in cystic fibrosis, TOBI
   d. Treatment of influenza in adults and children age 5 years and older, Relenza
8. Respirgard II
9. The Respirgard II should be powered with a flow rate of 5 to 7 L/min from a 50-psi source.
10. 1, 2
11. True
12. Cough
13. 20 mg/ml or 2% solution
14. The filters on the exhalation side of the patient circuit and proper functioning of the exhalation valve of the ventilator
15. Short half-life of 1–2 hours in respiratory secretions
16.
   a. Skin irritation
   b. Reduced pulmonary function
   c. Equipment malfunction due to drug precipitate
17.
   a. Children with bronchopulmonary dysplasia (BPD) and who are less than 2 years old
   b. Children less than 2 years of age and who have a history of premature birth (<35 weeks of gestation)
18. Intravenously (IV)
19. November, April
20. Premature
21. Intramuscular
22.
   a. To treat and prevent early colonization with *P. aeruginosa*
   b. To maintain present lung function and to reduce the rate of deterioration
23. False: It should be taken after all other therapies are finished.
24. False: They should not be mixed.
25. Yes: PARI-LC Plus and DeVilbiss Pulmo-Aide compressor
26. True
27. 10, 12
28. 5, 10
29. False
30. True

31. True
32. True
33. False: Especially if the patient has COPD or asthma

**NBRC-type Questions**

1. c
2. d
3. b
4. b
5. d
6. b
7. a
8. b
9. c
10. a
11. d
12. a
13. c
14. b
15. c

**Case Study**

1. Pretreatment of this patient with a bronchodilator!
2. No: Pentamidine should be delivered with a Respirgard II nebulizer system, which comes complete with expiratory filter and one-way valves.
3.
   a. Stop nebulization if the patient removes the mouthpiece
   b. Screen patient for TB
   c. Avoid exposure if you're pregnant or nursing
   d. Administer the treatment in a room with at least six air changes per hour (negative-pressure room)
   e. Use universal precautions.
4. Conjunctivitis and bronchospasm

## CHAPTER 14

1. Antimicrobials
2. Synergy
3. Antibiotics
4. Antagonism
5. Gram stain
6. Purple, pink
7. Acid-fast
8.
   a. 1, 4
   b. 2, 3, 4
   c. 3
   d. 2
   e. 1, 6
9. Kill, inhibit
10. Synergistically
11. Clinical assessment
12. Cell wall
13. Fourth generation
14. Broad-spectrum
15. True
16. Tobramycin

17.
   a. Gentamicin
   b. Tobramycin
18. Protein synthesis
19. Erythromycin
20. Telithromycin
21. Methicillin-resistant *Staphylococcus aureus* (MRSA)
22. 6 to 12
23. Aerosolization
24. Amphotericin
25.
   a. Immunocompromised patients with acquired immunodeficiency syndrome (AIDS)
   b. Cancer patients receiving chemotherapy
   c. Patients undergoing organ transplantation.
26. Replication

## NBRC-type Questions

1. b
2. a
3. d
4. d
5. b
6. d
7. a
8. b
9. c
10. d
11. d
12. a
13. a
14. d
15. d

## Case Study

1. Because the patient may be unreliable and/or noncompliant, the following treatment regimen is recommended: isoniazid, rifampin, pyrazinamide, and ethambutol plus vitamin $B_6$ daily for 2 weeks, then two or three times per week for 6 weeks. After that, isoniazid and rifampin plus vitamin $B_6$ should be taken two or three times per week for 6 months.
2. Streptomycin
3. This is a difficult question, but worth thinking about. He may comply, and then again he may not. If Mr. Green gets well, he could then return to New Orleans; a possible motivating factor. But in reality this may or may not be important to him. What's important to remember, however, is that you probably have no idea what it's like to be Mr. Green, so make no assumptions. He may be able to show up at a clinic, pick up his medications, and get a free meal. Ideally, it would be helpful to find him a better place to live, removing him from the environment where he got TB. It's also very important to tell Mr. Green that a noncompliant TB patient can be arrested.

## CHAPTER 15

1. Antihistamines
2. Flu
3. Stimulant expectorants
4. Expectorant
5. Common cold
6. Mucolytic expectorants
7. Antitussives
8.
   1. b
   2. a
   3. b
   4. b
   5. a
   6. b
   7. a
9.
   a. Sympathomimetics
   b. Antihistamines
   c. Expectorants
   d. Antitussives
10.
   a. Sympathomimetics, to decongest
   b. Antihistamines, to dry secretions
   c. Expectorants, to increase mucus clearance
   d. Antitussives, to suppress the cough reflex
11. Decongestant
12.
   a. Antihistamine—block bronchial smooth muscle constriction caused by histamine
   b. Sedative—antihistamines are absorbed into the brain
   c. Anticholinergic—upper airway drying
13. The airway drying may have a detrimental effect because secretion clearance is decreased.
14.
   a. Vagal gastric reflex stimulation
   b. Absorption into respiratory glands to directly increase mucus production
   c. Topical stimulation with inhaled volatile agents
15. Water
16.
   a. Reflex irritation of the bronchi
   b. Increased secretion clearance as a result of coughing
17. Codeine or hydrocodone
18. True
19. False
20. True
21.
   a. Tremor
   b. Tachycardia
   c. Hypertension
22.
   a. Drowsiness
   b. Impaired responses
   c. Drying of secretions
23. Questionable effectiveness; try water
24. Should never be used to suppress productive coughs

1. a
2. b
3. c
4. c
5. d
6. d
7. c
8. c
9. b
10. d
11. d
12. c
13. b
14. a
15. b

## Case Study

1. He has the classic symptoms of a cold.
2. Just like mom always said: rest, plenty of fluids, and perhaps an antihistamine for the runny nose.
3. If his temperature is normal, he's not lethargic, and he doesn't complain of a headache, he's still got a cold. If he does develop a dry, nonproductive cough add a cough suppressant (or antitussive, if you want to impress the pharmacist) to your list. The antitussive will also help him rest without being awakened by coughing. That way the little dear can get his strength back to hassle you in just a few short days!

## CHAPTER 16

1. b
2. a
3. e
4. c
5. d
6. Autosomal recessive
7. True
8. $\alpha_1$-Antitrypsin
9. Neutrophil elastase is held in check by $\alpha_1$-antitrypsin. If there's a deficiency in $\alpha_1$-antitrypsin, neutrophil elastase "burns through" alveolar walls and the result is emphysema.
10. Prolastin
11. Nicotine replacement therapy is initiated to replace the nicotine lost with smoking cessation.
12. The nicotine inhaler delivers less nicotine than the other nicotine systems, but simulates a cigarette and gives oral gratification.
13. True
14. True
15. Nicotine
16. Pulmonary
17. Selective
18. >34
19. 20
20. Nitrogen dioxide, methemoglobin
21. Before

22. False: Blood should be drawn more frequently than every other day.
23. True
24. False: Always start with the most minimal dose; 20 ppm is a common dose.
25. True
26. False: It is inactivated before reaching the systemic circulation.
27. True
28. Hemoglobin
29. Nitrate
30. Dilation, ventilation–perfusion
31. Bronchospasm
32.
    a. Smokers
    b. patients with uncontrolled lung disease
33. Immediately before meals

## NBRC-type Questions

1. a
2. c
3. b
4. c
5. d
6. a
7. a
8. a
9. b
10. d
11. a
12. d
13. a
14. c
15. c

## Case Study

1. Emphasize that she should continue to make time for your classes. Smoking cessation is accomplished on many levels, using behavior modification, group counseling, and education. Because she is such a public presence, chewing gum, inhaling a spray several times a day, taking lozenges, or using a nicotine inhaler would be too conspicuous! Recommend the transdermal patch (as long as she has no history of cardiovascular disease).
2. The most common reason for this occurrence is that she is not alternating skin sites. Suggest that she do this and see if this takes care of the problem.
3. Yes: Suggest that she begin with the highest dose (21 mg, equal to a half-pack per day) and gradually taper to a lower dose. This should be accomplished in no more than 3 months. Caution her not to smoke while she is wearing the patch. Educate her as to what withdrawal symptoms she can expect. Let her know that they will pass and teach her some coping techniques. Make sure she alternates the site of her patches so that she isn't bothered by skin irritation.
4. Bupropion (Zyban) is an antidepressant and nonnicotine medication that can help aid in smoking cessation. She can take this drug as well as continue

with the transdermal patch. Tell her that groups receiving both Zyban and the nicotine patch had a higher cessation rate than those using just the nicotine patch; this may pick up her spirits. Suggest that she try it for 7 weeks, and that if it doesn't work she may discontinue it. Consider placing the patient on varenicline (Chantix). Chantix works best if the patient sets a quit date and then starts taking the drug 1 week before the quit date.

## CHAPTER 17

1. b
2. i
3. d
4. e
5. h
6. a
7. c
8. j
9. f
10. g
11. a. The therapy should be reasonable and safe; b. Parameters used for monitoring during therapy should be predetermined; c. The drug is prescribed according to the standards of care.
12. Avoidance of systemic factors that can affect oral or injectable drug therapy

|  | Neonate | Adult |
|---|---|---|
| 13. Tracheal length | 5-6 cm | 10-12 cm |
| 14. Tidal volume | 6 ml/kg | 6 ml/kg |
| 15. Minute ventilation | 200-300 ml/kg/min | 6 L/min |
| 16. Respiratory rate | 30-40/min | 12-14/min |
| 17. Inspiratory flow rate | ≤100 ml/s | ≈500 ml/s |

18. Any three of the following are correct: smaller diameter lower airways, smaller tidal volume, breathing pattern, small inspiratory flow rate, small endotracheal tube
19. True
20. False: The emitted dose is less than the nominal dose.
21. 1%, 2.5%
22. Deposition
23. Any three of the following is correct: low tidal volume, low vital capacity, short respiratory cycle, low inspiratory flow rate
24. Small enough to allow drug inhalation with a few breaths with tidal volumes <50 ml.
25. a
26. b
27. a
28. b
29. a
30. Small airways blocked by secretions, poor development of smooth muscle
31. SVN with mask, MDI with ETT
32. Breath-actuated MDI, DPI, and MDI
33. MDI with reservoir
34. MDI with reservoir/mask
35. 50%
36. The patient must be able to generate a minimal flow rate of 60 L/min, which is difficult or impossible for small children.
37. Any of the following three is correct: unexpected increases in volume and pressure, bias flow interfering with patient-triggered modes of ventilation, unexpected increases in positive end-expiratory pressure (PEEP), variable fraction of inspired oxygen ($F_{I_{O2}}$).
38. Manual

**NBRC-type Questions**

1. c
2. d
3. d
4. b
5. d
6. a
7. c
8. d
9. b
10. a
11. b
12. c
13. d
14. a
15. d
16. d

**Case Study**

1. SVN, MDI with spacer and mask, MDI with endotracheal tube
2. You could choose either an SVN or MDI with spacer and mask as long as you provide good reasons. An SVN would typically be chosen, based only on the child's age. Most 18-month-olds will tolerate a mask held loosely against their face as long as you're making a game of it. Unfortunately, this will reduce the amount of drug the infant receives. The same rule also applies in pediatrics. With an SVN there are many more chances (breaths) to deliver the medication; with an MDI, you've got only two or three chances.
3. Have one of the parents give the treatment.
4. Because of the potential problems associated with in-line nebulization, such as excessive pressure or volume, altered $F_{I_{O2}}$, triggering problems, and excessive PEEP, MDI treatment placed in-line would be best.

## CHAPTER 18

1. c
2. g
3. i
4. h
5. b

6. d

7. a

8. j

9. e

10. l

11. f

12. k

13. Depolarizing agents bind to acetylcholine receptors and cause a sustained postsynaptic membrane depolarization. Nondepolarizing agents produce paralysis and muscle weakness by competing with acetylcholine for binding at the acetylcholine receptors.

14. Succinylcholine

15. Voluntary, involuntary

16. Acetylcholine (ACh)

17. Acetylcholinesterase (AChE)

18. Depolarization, repolarization

19. The patient has drooping eyelids and is unable to move the head.

20. There is diaphragmatic function as seen by movement of the abdomen.

21. (1) Maintaining a patent airway and (2) maintaining appropriate ventilation, because nondepolarizing agents cause apnea

22. Anticholinesterase, such as neostigmine

23. Pyridostigmine

24.
   a. Tachycardia
   b. Increased salivation

25. *d*-Tubocurarine

26. Pancuronium

27. Intubation

28. Fasciculations

29.
   a. Histamine release
   b. Hypertension
   c. Tachycardia

30. Nosocomial pneumonia

31. Aspiration

32. Sedation and analgesia

33. Amnestic

34. True

35.
   a. Small, rapidly moving muscles such as the eyelids
   b. Face
   c. Neck;
   d. Extremities
   e. Abdomen
   f. Intercostals
   g. Diaphragm

36.
   a. Hand grip strength
   b. The ability to lift the head off the bed for 5 seconds

37. True

## NBRC-type Questions

1. a

2. a

3. d

4. b

5. b

6. a

7. b

8. c

9. d

10. b

11. c

12. d

13. c

14. a

## Case Study

1. Succinylcholine is a good choice because it takes effect quickly and wears off in 10 to 15 minutes. This will give you enough time to intubate and stabilize the endotracheal tube without leaving him paralyzed unnecessarily long.

2. Use a nondepolarizing agent for long-term ventilator care. Vecuronium is a good choice because it has minimal effects on the cardiovascular system and histamine release is not an issue.

3. *d*-Tubocurarine, because it is the most potent releaser of histamine.

4. A sedative and, if the patient is not already receiving it, pain medication.

5. Suction the patient as needed, using sterile technique. Keep the head of the bed raised.

6. His abdomen moves, indicating diaphragmatic use.

## CHAPTER 19

1. c

2. d

3. f

4. g

5. a

6. e

7. b

8. j

9. i

10. h

11. $CO = HR \times SV = 80 \times 70 = 5.6$ L/min

12. Preload

13.
   a. Systemic vascular resistance
   b. Vascular volume

14. $MAP = (2DBP + SBP)/3 = [(120 \times 2) + 90]/3 = 330/3 = 110$ mmHg

15. Central venous pressure

16. 5-12 mmHg

17. 10-12 mmHg

18. 5-7 L/min

19. 800-1440 (dyn • sec • cm$^{-5}$)

20. a

21. b

22. b

23. a

24. b

25. b

26. a
27. Vasoconstriction
28. Cardiac
29. Septic
30. True
31. True
32. Heart failure
33.
   a. SA node
   b. AV node
   c. Bundle of His
   d. Ventricular bundle branches
   e. Purkinje fibers
34. Fibrillation and flutter
35. Tachycardia
36. Ventricular
37. Bronchoconstriction
38. Ventricular
39. Calcium channel
40. Vasoconstriction of the coronary and cerebral vasculature, increasing blood flow to these areas
41. Potent vasoconstrictor
42. Chronotropic effect on the heart
43. Increase arterial pH above 7.2. Adequate ventilation must be present to remove the carbon dioxide produced, otherwise a continual reduction in pH will continue.
44. Prolong conduction time often implemented in the management of torsades de pointes.
45. When IV access is difficult or impossible
46. The four agents can be remembered by the acronym LEAN: a. Lidocaine; b. Epinephrine; c. Atropine; d. Naloxone
47. False: Chest compressions should cease.
48. True
49. True
50. True

**NBRC-type Questions**

1. c
2. d
3. a
4. b
5. d
6. a
7. c
8. b
9. d
10. c
11. d
12. d
13. c
14. b
15. d

**Case Study**

1. Hypovolemic/hemorrhagic
2.
   a. BP, decreased. Her BP is probably 70/30
   b. Heart rate, increased. Her heart rate is probably 156 beats/min. The body increases its heart rate to increase cardiac output (remember that heart rate × stroke volume = cardiac output)
   c. CVP, decreased. Her CVP is most likely <5 mmHg
   d. CO, decreased. Her cardiac output is most likely <5 L/min
   e. SVR, increased. The systemic vascular resistance increases in an effort to maintain blood pressure and cardiac output. Therefore her SVR is most likely >1440 dyn • s • cm$^{-5}$.
3. The lidocaine should be administered through the ETT.
4. She is now normovolemic. Her blood pressure would indicate her systemic vascular resistance has returned to normal and her vascular volume is increased. These two are the major components of blood pressure. Her cardiac output is increased. Nice work.

## CHAPTER 20

1. c
2. h
3. k
4. r
5. e
6. p
7. n
8. d
9. a
10. f
11. b
12. g
13. q
14. l
15. i
16. m
17. j
18. o
19. 120/80
20. True
21. Hypertensive crisis
22. Renin–angiotensin–aldosterone
23.
   a. Reduction in peripheral arterial resistance
   b. Increase in cardiac output
   c. Little or no change in heart rate
   d. Increase in renal blood flow and unchanged glomerular filtration rate (GFR)
24. True
25.
   a. Angina
   b. Arrhythmia
   c. Hypertension
26. It means that verapamil reduces the heart rate and the contractility of the heart
27. False: The majority occur during the morning hours.

28.
   a. Bronchospasm
   b. Bronchial obstruction
   c. Wheezing
   d. Dyspnea
   e. Cough
   f. Exacerbation of previously stable asthma or chronic airway obstruction
29.
   a. Thiazides
   b. Potassium-sparing agents
30. By affecting both cardiac output and peripheral resistance; they are negative inotropes and chronotropes.
31. It exerts a direct action on vascular smooth muscle.
32.
   a. Chest tightness
   b. Pressure
   c. Burning sensation (indigestion) radiating to left shoulder and jaw
33. By vasodilation of coronary arteries
34. Sublingually
35. Every 5 minutes until the pain is relieved. If the pain is not relieved in 15 minutes, seek emergency care.
36. The treatment of chronic angina patients who do not respond to other antianginal drugs.
37.
   a. Prevention of thromboembolism
   b. Prevention of pulmonary embolism
38. True
39. Aspirin, especially at high doses, can induce or exacerbate asthma and dyspnea in patients with COPD.
40. True
41. True

**NBRC-type Questions**

1. a
2. b
3. d
4. c
5. c
6. a
7. d
8. a
9. c
10. d
11. b
12. c
13. a
14. d
15. b

**Case Study**

1. Angina may present as chest tightness, pressure, or a burning sensation (indigestion) and may radiate to the left shoulder and jaw. Her heart rate probably is high, which is consuming more oxygen. Her discomfort is from coronary artery vasoconstriction.

2. Yes: Open containers should be discarded after 6 months.
3. Sublingual nitroglycerin has an onset of action of minutes and a duration of action of 30 minutes.
4. Give her another nitroglycerin pill.
5. Call 911 and get to a hospital.

**CHAPTER 21**

1. b
2. d
3. f
4. a
5. j
6. h
7. c
8. e
9. g
10. i
11. Nephrons
12. Glomerular filtration rate
13. Atrial natriuretic peptide
14. Antidiuretic hormone
15. Renin–angiotension system
16. Hypochloremia, hypokalemia
17. Cerebral edema
18. Water, NaCl
19. Metabolic alkalosis (remember: $CO_2 + H_2O \leftrightarrow HCO_3^- + H^+$. CAI prevents the normal breakdown of carbonic acid and, therefore, decreases bicarbonate reabsorption)
20. Potassium
21. Diuresis
22. Vasodilating
23. 20, doubled
24. Hypertension
25. Loop, thiazide
26.
   a. Hypovolemia
   b. Electrolyte imbalance
   c. Acid–base imbalance
27.
   a. Potassium level < 3.0 mEq/L
   b. Patients with history of heart disease or symptoms of low potassium
   c. Patients taking digitalis
28. Hyperglycemia
29. Furosemide
30. Thiazide diuretics
31. Potassium-sparing diuretics
32. Carbonic anhydrase inhibitors
33. Osmotic diuretics
34. Loop diuretics

**NBRC-type Questions**

1. d
2. a
3. d
4. d
5. b

6. d
7. b
8. a
9. c
10. b
11. c
12. d
13. b
14. d
15. c

## Case Study

1. Change the nasal cannula to either a Venturi mask at 50% or to a nonrebreathing mask to increase her $SpO_2$.
2. CHF
3. Loop diuretic: Lasix
4. Doubling the dose until diuresis occurs
5. Potassium and chloride replacement
6. Metabolic alkalosis
7. Potassium and chloride replacement

## CHAPTER 22

1. f
2. c
3. b
4. i
5. a
6. d
7. h
8. k
9. e
10. g
11. j
12.
    a. Midbrain
    b. Pons
    c. Medulla
13. Parkinson disease
14.
    a. Norepinephrine
    b. Dopamine
    c. Acetylcholine
15. Serotonin, norepinephrine
16. Mood stabilizer
17. Bipolar
18. Dopamine
19. Cholinesterase inhibitors
20.
    a. Thiopental, anesthetic induction
    b. Pentobarbital, hypnotic
    c. Phenobarbital, seizure control
21. Difficulty sleeping
22. Delirium tremens (DTs)
23. True
24. Analgesics
25. True
26. Aspirin

27. Aspirin reduces inflammation, whereas Tylenol does not.
28. An opioid analgesic: Morphine, codeine, and Demerol are common opioid receptor agonists.
29. Naloxone (Narcan) is one example of an opioid antagonist.
30. False: It may help with bronchodilation and suppress the cough by reducing irritation of the lung.
31. Heart rate, blood pressure
32. Three
33. Resuscitation equipment
34.
    a. Dedicated monitoring assistant
    b. Pulse oximetry
    c. IV access
    d. Blood pressure measurement every 15 minutes
35. Caffeine
36. True
37. True
38. True

## NBRC-type Questions

1. d
2. c
3. d
4. d
5. b
6. a
7. c
8. c
9. a
10. c
11. c
12. b
13. a
14. b
15. c
16. d
17. a
18. b
19. c
20. c
21. b
22. c
23. b
24. a
25. c

## Case Study

1. Respiratory stimulants do not treat respiratory failure or provide a sustained improvement in respiratory failure. Mr. Jones has an acute on chronic respiratory failure. He requires ventilation assistance to rest his respiratory muscles and provide ventilatory improvement. Placing the patient on BiPAP (bilevel positive airway pressure) therapy or mechanical ventilation would be the correct suggestion.
2. Resuscitation equipment should be at the bedside in case the patient's airway is compromised.

3. Pulse oximetry, blood pressure, ventilation, heart rate, respiratory rate
4. Naloxone (Narcan) is a specific antagonist that will reverse the effects of respiratory depression brought on by the opioid.

5. Caffeine is used therapeutically to treat apnea in premature infants. This is especially important when the infant is placed on CPAP, where it is essential that the infant maintain spontaneous respirations.